"This book is a generous and accessible call to health and wholeness for individuals and society. Ward Ewing has graced it with honest anecdotes that help the reader identify the power of spirituality in their lives with or without religion. He doesn't pull any punches, and there is no condescension. *Twelve Steps to Religionless Spirituality* is full of experience, strength, and hope."

—CLARK BERGE
SSF, former minister general for the Society of St. Francis

"Ward Ewing brings to us a lifetime of experience being attentive to human longing, angst, tenderness, and has seen again and again our capacity for transformation. One thing is clear: For all of our differences we seek and long for the same thing. To be seen, loved, accepted. . . . Ward draws our attention to the remarkable work of AA and its understanding of the human condition. Whether you know the twelve steps by heart or are unfamiliar with them and didn't think they applied to you, this book is an important read. It reminds us of our capacity for honesty and trust, compassion and regard, love and reconciliation. That is the healing work of AA. That is our healing work together. Our hope is in us."

—MARIANNE W. BORG
Widow of theologian Marcus J. Borg and retired Episcopal priest

TWELVE STEPS
TO RELIGIONLESS
SPIRITUALITY

To Marilyn Wilson
With gratitude for your friendship

Ward B. Ewing
2 December, 2021

TWELVE STEPS TO RELIGIONLESS SPIRITUALITY

The Power of Spirituality with or without God

WARD B. EWING

CASCADE *Books* · Eugene, Oregon

TWELVE STEPS TO RELIGIONLESS SPIRITUALITY
The Power of Spirituality with or without God

Cascade Books
An Imprint of Wipf and Stock Publishers
199 W. 8th Ave., Suite 3
Eugene, OR 97401

www.wipfandstock.com

PAPERBACK ISBN: 978-1-7252-7902-5
HARDCOVER ISBN: 978-1-7252-7903-2
EBOOK ISBN: 978-1-7252-7904-9

Cataloguing-in-Publication data:

Names: Ewing, Ward B.
Title: Twelve steps to religionless spirituality : the power of spirituality with or without God / Ward B. Ewing.
Description: Eugene, OR: Cascade Publications, 2021 | Includes bibliographical references.
Identifiers: ISBN 978-1-7252-7902-5 (paperback) | ISBN 978-1-7252-7903-2 (hardcover) | ISBN 978-1-7252-7904-9 (ebook)
Subjects: LCSH: Spiritual life. | Twelve-step programs—Religious aspects—Christianity.
Classification: HV5186 .E50 2021 (paperback) | HV5186 (ebook)

09/03/21

The brief excerpts from Alcoholics Anonymous World Services, Inc. ("A.A.W.S.") and the A.A. Grapevine, Inc. copyrighted material are reprinted with permission. Permission to reprint these excerpts does not mean that A.A.W.S. and the Grapevine has reviewed or approved the contents of this publication, or that it necessarily agrees with the views expressed herein. A.A. is a program of recovery from alcoholism only – use of these excerpts in connection with programs and activities which are patterned after A.A., but which address other problems, or in any other non A.A. context, does not imply otherwise. Additionally, while A.A. is a spiritual program, A.A. is not a religious program. Thus, A.A. is not affiliated or allied with any sect, denomination, or specific religious belief.

Stories and commentary from *Experiencing Spirituality* and *The Spirituality of Imperfection* are reprinted by permission from Katherine Ketcham and Linda Kurtz, the widow of Ernest Kurtz.

I dedicate this volume to my friends in the church
and to my friends in the Fellowship of Alcoholics Anonymous.
Together they have taught me much and nurtured my spiritual growth.

I also dedicate this to my loving wife.
We celebrated our fifty-third anniversary this year.
Her support and love are simply the most important part of my life.

Contents

Preface

OUR AGE IS, ABOVE all, a time of change. Advances in science and technology, the proliferation of capitalism and free markets, increasing urbanization and globalization, the extension of the expected human life span, social media and the ability to choose the news one accepts, multiculturalism, and large immigration movements have led to increasing polarization and conflict in our society and our world. We are largely in denial about the destruction coming as a result of climate change. Divisive partisan politics have damaged our ability to work together to resolve differences. The politicized approach to the COVID-19 pandemic and the continued struggles of racism made visible by the Black Lives Matter movement are among the most recent events reflecting this polarization and resulting conflict.

In this changing world the search for truth is often lost. Partisan differences have led many to believe that no one is providing factual information, and everyone simply makes up his or her own narrative. People become so invested in their personal perspective that facts suggesting a different view are ignored. Everything from politics to religion to sports has been revealed as corrupted or corruptible. And every mismanaged war, failed hurricane response, botched investigation, and doping scandal furthers this view.

This deep polarization is also evident in the spiritual realm. The religious institutions that have in the past provided unity, value, and direction have diminished in authority and influence. In their place we find conflicts between the traditionally religious, liberal Christians, evangelicals, fundamentalists, Jews, Muslims, and those who see themselves as spiritual and not religious, as well as secularists, agnostics, and atheists. We face a curious phenomenon that while institutional religion in North America and Europe is in decline people seem attracted to "spirituality."

The need for dialogue, openness, and tolerance cannot be overstated. Many scholars in the fields of sociology, psychology, and theology seek to articulate the implications of these cultural changes. Using new insights and ancient traditions they seek to develop a new consensus that will provide a basis for civil conversation and reconciliation. I write in the hope that insights from the spirituality of Twelve-Step recovery programs may be added to this conversation. Because Twelve-Step spirituality is not studied in academia and is largely unknown outside Twelve-Step recovery groups, it is not part of these debates and is not viewed as an important resource. Twelve-Step spirituality is a different way for understanding truth and spirituality and has much to contribute to these conversations. This book, based on my experience as a nonalcoholic religious leader who found his primary spiritual program in the Twelve Steps and the Fellowship of Alcoholics Anonymous, seeks to add perspectives from this experience to this conversation.

In the midst of our polarized world, Alcoholics Anonymous has since its founding been remarkably inclusive. Christians, Jews, Muslims, as well as the nonreligious, atheists, and agnostics can be found in the rooms of A.A. Members include people from many races, including Caucasian, African, Hispanic, Asian, Native American, and more. Male and female, gay and straight, conservative and liberal—all are welcome and have been since the first years of the program. The book *Alcoholics Anonymous* has been translated into sixty-seven languages, including American Sign Language (ASL) and Navajo. All communication from the General Service Office of A.A. is in French, Spanish, and English. A.A. groups are found in approximately 180 nations. Insights into how Alcoholics Anonymous and other Twelve-Step-based programs work with such diversity may be helpful as we seek to mend the polarization of our current culture.

This ability to include such diversity comes in part because Twelve-Step spirituality is dramatically different from the typical religious faith. Members are not asked to commit to any theology or doctrine. The God of our understanding is defined by each individual based on whatever power enabled the person to recover from addiction. The focus is on what has worked for other alcoholics, and what has worked is shared through the telling of personal stories. As members hear the stories, they seek to identify with those parts they have in common. The result of this approach is a strong community that is inclusive and welcomes all who desire to stop drinking. This works for atheists and agnostics, secularists and free thinkers, Christians, Jews, Muslims, and those who have no religious affiliation (often referred to as "nones").

To be human is to be a spiritual being. The question we all face is: How do we grow spiritually? This question is one we face as members of religious organizations that struggle with the meaning of faith in our secular world. It is also faced by those who are not part of religious organizations, as well as by those who refer to themselves as atheists, agnostics, and free thinkers. I believe the pragmatic understanding of spirituality that is found in the Twelve Steps contains understandings that provide support and transformation for all who seek spiritual renewal. The spirituality of the Steps provides a different perspective on religion and spirituality and offers a way for spiritual growth for many in our current secular culture. As illustrated in the Fellowship of Alcoholics Anonymous, we see that this pragmatic, spiritual program can heal, empower, and restore relationships for a great diversity of people from a wide multiplicity of backgrounds. Our secular society, where people profess that they are spiritual but not religious, could learn much from the experience of those in recovery. Just as A.A. includes such dramatic diversity in a supportive community, perhaps we can learn ways to begin to bridge the division and polarization that so characterize our age.

I share this essay with the hope that some pieces may provide insights to others, as they have to me, to strengthen their lives and their wills in service to others. For the nones who seek spiritual growth outside religious institutions, Twelve-Step spirituality challenges them to become serious about transformation, community, and service. For religious leaders and active members in church and synagogue, Twelve-Step spirituality challenges them to move from concern about correct doctrine and institutional preservation to strengthen the emphasis on the power of spirituality to transform people's lives and build communities of compassion. For members of A.A. who have encouraged me to write, I hope this book will strengthen their commitment to continue in the process of spiritual progress.

I am an ordained minister in the Episcopal Church. I served congregations in Memphis and Bristol, Tennessee; Jacksonville, Florida; Louisville, Kentucky; and Buffalo, New York before I was elected Dean and President of the General Theological Seminary in New York City. My ministry has been varied but always included a strong focus on education.

I have been fortunate as one who does not suffer from the disease of alcoholism to be deeply involved with Alcoholics Anonymous for the past forty-five years. I attend open meetings from time to time. I am a member of our denomination's program for education and support. I have sponsored multiple education events for clergy and for congregations. Recently I have served as a Trustee on the General Service Board of Alcoholics Anonymous for the United States and Canada. From 2009 to 2013, I served as Chair of the Board. The Twelve Steps of Alcoholics Anonymous have served as my primary spiritual program for the past forty years. My ministry and my life have been strengthened and enriched by this spiritual program.

This book comes in response to requests from members of A.A. and from members of congregations where I have served. In particular, participants in two weekend retreats I led for men in A.A.—St. Martin's Retreat Group in Mendham, New Jersey and The Promises Weekend in Tahlequah, Oklahoma—encouraged me to share my experience with a wider audience. My experience with A.A., my service in the church, and my personal reflections on Twelve-Step spirituality and leadership lead me to believe there are many who may benefit from sharing this experience.

* * *

I begin expressing gratitude by giving thanks for my wife, Jenny, who has supported my desire to write even when it has intruded on our retirement. After fifty-three years she is still the one. The Promises Weekend represented a definite change for me from considering if I should write to beginning the process of putting some thoughts on paper. Deborah K., a member of the A.A. Fellowship, PhD medical researcher, and dear friend, more than anyone else has encouraged and supported me in developing this book, serving as my primary critical assistant. Other support has come from Caroline V., Stuart H., Howard B., and Robert G.—clergy who are also members of Twelve-Step Fellowships. Ernest Kurtz and Katherine Ketcham in different ways have been supportive and helpful, as has Terry Bedient, who succeeded me as Chair of the General Service Board. I was privileged to be a keynote speaker at the first International Conference for Atheists, Agnostics, and Free Thinkers in A.A.; the leadership of Joe C. and others in this group have been important to me. And I have been deeply influenced by the work of the Rev. Dr. Marcus Borg on the historical Jesus and the sharing of his personal faith story. The General Service Office of Alcoholics Anonymous and the office for A.A. Grapevine have been supportive and very helpful. The material available through www.aa.org and www.aagrapevine.org is voluminous.

I want to be clear that I write to share my experience; this book is not part of any official understandings about Alcoholics Anonymous. Many members of A.A. may well take exception to some of what I write. The diversity in A.A. is dramatic, particularly when matters of spirituality and religion are concerned. The Fellowship, which is found in countries around the world, represents a variety of cultures and religious experience. My experience is just that—my experience. In no way should this book be seen as an official expression of A.A. spirituality.

For those unfamiliar with the Twelve Steps and the Twelve Traditions, copies are found along with the Preamble in Appendix A at the end of this book. I have also included in Appendix B a brief chronology of the early years of A.A., as several references to this history are in the text.

The Very Rev. Ward B. Ewing DD
Summer 2020

CHAPTER 1

Introduction

Willie

WILLIE WALKED INTO MY office.

"You're the spiritual expert, right?" he said without the usual "Hello."

I was the vicar of a small congregation in Louisville, Kentucky; Willie was a member of the congregation. Several years before, in order to learn about alcoholism, I began attending open meetings of Alcoholics Anonymous. Willie was also a member of that Fellowship.

I did not respond to Willie's opening statement; he continued.

"I am out of touch with God. The last time I was out of touch with my Higher Power, I drank. If I drink again, I may die. I need you to put me back in touch with God."

He had my attention. I stopped what I was doing. We talked. I had enough sense to know I could not put him back in touch with God. I also knew if I were to be helpful I would have to know a lot more about the struggles those addicted to alcohol have with theology and personal issues and how this all fits together with sobriety. So we talked. And we talked again the next day and decided to put together a small group composed of members of A.A. who had at least five years of sobriety and who would like to discuss the "spiritual issues" in their lives. I was to be part of this group.

A.A. is a spiritual program. It is not religious. There is no theology, no official liturgy, no professional leaders, no doctrine, no criteria for membership other than the desire to stop drinking. The spirituality of A.A. is based on experience, not doctrine. The fundamental spiritual experience that enables sobriety is the movement from being self-directed—I am strong, I can control my drinking, I need to control you—to being directed by a power greater than self. Many in the Fellowship understand that power greater than self as God. However, to avoid religiosity, from the beginning, as the Steps were being developed and the book *Alcoholics Anonymous* was being written, the terms "God as we understand him," or more simply "Higher Power," were used to refer to this power that enables the alcoholic to control his or her drinking. Members' understandings of God vary from a traditional theistic God to the power found in the support of the Fellowship ("Group of Drunks" or "Good Orderly Direction"). In most meetings, there is an active avoidance of doctrinal-based terminology, as members are aware that this narrows effectiveness to those that believe (or do not believe) in a specific manner. Indeed many find the spirituality of the Steps works for them because of the generous latitude that allows development of their own private definitions in their own small quiet corner—free of judgment, free of insistent conformity, free of rules.

Many come to A.A. bearing loads of resentment and guilt that have been reinforced by churches that are all too ready to advise, imply judgment, or condemn outright. Sometimes this judgment is a direct condemnation from some preacher or church member; sometimes it is a kind of indirect moralism that declares that anyone who drinks or drinks too much is weak; sometimes it is a kind of shunning that excludes the drinker from the "Christian" fellowship. However the judgment comes, to the person still struggling with addiction to alcohol, it is fuel for resentment, guilt, and despair. Few attend their first meeting of A.A. with a healthy faith. The newcomer may easily be turned off when they hear talk of God or faith.

As a result, though god-language is often heard in A.A. meetings, issues of spiritual experience or theological challenges like the problem of evil or the nature of prayer and meditation are rarely discussed. Not surprisingly, after a person has been a member for a few years such problems of faith may emerge. The initial "coming to believe there is a power greater than self that can restore sanity" (Step 2) may be eroded when the sense of crisis diminishes. Our little group provided a place where those who shared the experience of addiction could also share their faith, their doubts, their struggles with institutional religion, and their experience of a Higher Power.

Our little group also changed my life. We met every Tuesday afternoon until I moved away from Louisville five years later. I am certain I gained more from them than they from me. They gave me a spiritual program that has been central for my life ever since. Just as the members of A.A. needed a place to share their spiritual experiences, their doubts, and their concerns, I too needed a place where I could be honest about myself. Our mutual need made this group truly collaborative. In my teenage years I substituted success for love with disastrous results of loneliness and depression. Despite the faith that saved my life, I continued to be an overly responsible workaholic. I struggled with the need to be in control and with the seduction of admiration and respect, when what I truly needed was to be known and loved. The members of the group brought a standard of honesty that I have rarely experienced outside of the A.A. Fellowship. No one cared about what one might share as long as he was trying to be as honest as possible. We were not confrontative with one another. But through the honest sharing, I began learning to let go and let God be in charge, to be more vulnerable about sharing my weaknesses, to listen and learn from folks whose lives were dramatically different from mine, and to see how my being overly responsible discouraged others from getting involved. This journey continues, but this group helped me set my understanding of ministry. I am less afraid of uncomfortable truth; I understand that hope is often related to failure; and that failure shared appropriately can be a strength for self and others. The strengths of my ministry have been in the development of collaborative communities and in nurturing the transformation possible through small group experiences. I also discovered after leaving Louisville as I put together my support group with other clergy, if a member of A.A. was in the group it was more honest, more focused on personal concerns, and less fearful of self-disclosure.

Clergy have a difficult time finding a group where they can be totally honest. Parishioners and society in general want clergy to be good—that is distinctly different from being honest. This isolation imposes much pressure with the result that some clergy end up violating their own standards for ethical behavior. Most clergy, however, simply endure the stress of their job quietly, faithfully, and stoically. The results are clergy burnout or lackadaisical, passive, dispassionate performance of ministry. It's not that clergy have mammoth amounts of unacceptable thoughts or actions to confess; it's the isolation and the expectations that add to the stress of dealing constantly with people. I, like many clergy, could share my thoughts and feelings with my wife, but that often placed her emotionally in a difficult place with parishioners. She should not have to bear all my frustration.

I am an ordained minister because the church by word and action taught me that I am loved by God. Even though I did not feel worthy, God loves and cares for me as I am. I cannot create my worth by my achievements. Rather to understand I have worth, all I must do is accept that love that is present all around me. The Twelve Steps have provided me a concrete spiritual program that has allowed me to grow and develop the faith the church had given me. Because of this group, the Steps, and the Fellowship of A.A., I have become more honest and more open to others (honestly recognizing we all have character defects). I am less concerned about getting credit and more able to ask for assistance. I am better at building collaboration, more able to deal with fear, and I comprehend the need for all of us to find personal transformation that leads to service to others. As a result I have a better marriage, I am a better father, and I have close friends.

I believe the Fellowship of A.A. provides a model that can inform our religious institutions and bring life-transforming power to our broken world. I share my experience in the church and in Twelve-Step spirituality as part of the ongoing conversations in Western culture regarding the possibilities of spiritual renewal, in the hope that these conversations will yield a blueprint for spirituality that anyone can embrace and grow spiritually.

Religion and Spirituality

It is not news to say that Western culture is becoming more and more secular. Western Europe, where Protestant Christianity originated and Catholicism has been based for most of its history, has become one of the world's most secular regions. Although the vast majority of adults say they were baptized, and a majority identify themselves as Christian, only 22 percent attend services at least monthly. In the United States the trend is more complicated. The fastest-growing category with regard to religious groups are the "nones"—those who say they have no religious affiliation—who now represent 23 percent of the population. However, 89 percent of US adults say they believe in God. About six in ten adults say they regularly feel a deep sense of "spiritual peace and well-being," and 46 percent of Americans say they experience a deep sense of "wonder about the universe." Some identify these figures as indicating that Americans are becoming less religious and more spiritual. The trends are clearly moving in the direction of nonaffiliation, as young people make up a majority of the "nones." As the older cohorts of adults pass away, they are being replaced by a new cohort of young adults who display far lower levels of attachment to organized religion than their parents' and grandparents' generations did when they were the same age.[1] This is a time of significant transition. If churches, synagogues, and mosques are to continue to provide personal support for individuals and cultural influence for society, we must develop a spirituality that is congruent with this changing culture.

Few terms are more loosely used in our culture than the terms "spiritual" and "spirituality." Many say they are "spiritual" but not "religious"; but to define "spiritual" as "not religious" is totally inadequate. We do not know what something is by saying it is not something else. Other people, on the other hand, often use the terms "spirituality" or "spiritual" to refer to religion. Certainly for the religious, spirituality is connected to religion. The next chapter discusses the meanings of "spiritual" and "spirituality," but I think it is important to make clear distinctions between religion and spirituality from the beginning.

Organized religion—I prefer the term institutionalized religion—has a set of beliefs that form a core theology. Most churches codify these beliefs into some kind of dogma or creed, even if they do not use the word "dogma." To support this structure of belief, institutionalized religion has an organizational structure, often hierarchical, dominated by the ordained clergy who represent those who truly know the belief system and the practice. There will be a regular, even regulated, style of worship with set prayers, expectations about sermons, and largely focused on the ordained leaders. And there are ethical implications based on the belief system—some "don'ts" and some "dos." (Don't swear, don't drink, don't lie; do support the church, do work hard.) When ethics becomes attached to a focus on guilt and repentance, this ethic seems to represent a program for perfection; we are less than acceptable if we fail. Generally these aspects of religion represent clear boundaries that define who the members are: who is in and who is out. And those who are in are asked to give financially to support the institution.

"Spiritual," on the other hand, is broad and inclusive. "Spiritual realities" represent all those things that affect our lives but which we cannot see or touch—things like love, resentment, hope, anger, peace, anxiety, serenity. Spiritual realities are present for all human beings. Spirituality has nothing to do with boundaries, with who is "in" and who is "out," or

---

1 These figures and additional information can be found at the Pew Research Center, www.pewforum.org/data.

with "in-groups" and "out-groups." Spiritual realities are difficult to teach intellectually; they are best shared not through doctrines but through the sharing of personal stories.

Without question the Twelve Steps lay out a spiritual program, but it is a spirituality based on experience, not doctrine. As the Big Book[2] says, "The spiritual life is not a theory. *We have to live it*" (83; italics original). Central in the spirituality of A.A. is mystery, not doctrine—mystery at the miracle of lives changed by following these simple principles.

Religionless Christianity

Perhaps the most creative Christian thinker in the twentieth century was the German theologian and martyr, Dietrich Bonhoeffer. While in prison for his opposition to the Third Reich and before his involvement in the plot to kill Hitler became known, Bonhoeffer wrote letters expressing some stimulating thoughts about what he called "religionless Christianity."[3]

The influence of Karl Barth in his early theological training had led him to reject "religion" as being the "most grandiose and subtle" of mankind's self-centered efforts to gain possession of the infinite. He had come to see in religion a particular department of culture, intent upon its own self-preservation. Relying upon privilege, concerned with being rich and powerful, when criticized, religion often took refuge in metaphysics that Bonhoeffer called "a flight from reality into convenient abstractions."[4]

"While Bonhoeffer's initial concern about religion reflected the position of Barth's neo-orthodoxy, in letters as early as 1931, following his return to Germany from the United States, he expressed his frustration that the Christian community seemed inert, almost indifferent, to the unparalleled economic situation of suffering and need. The failure of the church in Germany to take a stand against the influence and control of the Third Reich strengthened his conviction that institutional religion was unable to proclaim strongly the biblical and theological message. Beginning when Hitler came to power in 1933, through the ecumenical movement, the Council of Young Reformers, and as Director of the seminary for the

2. The book *Alcoholics Anonymous* is often referred to as the "Big Book." Because of the numerous citations from this book, instead of footnotes the page numbers will be included in the text (#).

3. Bosanquet, *Life and Death of Dietrich Bonhoeffer*, 257.

4. Bosanquet, *Life and Death of Dietrich Bonhoeffer*, 257.

Confessing Church, he actively opposed the nationalism and antisemitism of the Führer. His involvement in the resistance to Hitler and his imprisonment pushed him to look further at our world, a world that had ceased to be religious. Just a few phrases that were popularized from his letters indicate the creativity of his thought:

"Mankind come of age" describes his understanding that humankind as a whole has ceased to be religious. God is no longer needed as a solution to human problems, as human beings have "learned to deal with all questions of importance without recourse to 'the working hypothesis' called 'God.'"[5]

"God in the gaps" describes his understanding of how the churches sought to respond to science and secularity by asserting that God answers those problems we have not solved, such as death and guilt. He wrote, "[in contrast] I should like to speak of God not on the boundaries but at the center, not in weakness but in strength; and therefore not in death and guilt but in man's life and goodness."[6] "We are to find God in what we know, not in what we do not know."[7]

How are we, as people of faith, to live in this world come of age, he asked? We must repent from the religious perspective that seeks to get God to do our will and begin to seek first to do the divine will through the exercise of "ultimate honesty." Then we will "really live in the godless world without attempting to gloss over or explain its ungodliness in some religious way or other." Then we will share "in God's sufferings at the hands of a godless world" for God in his powerlessness allows "himself to be pushed out of the world on to the cross."[8] One learns to have faith only by living unreservedly in this world, for by "so doing we throw ourselves completely into the arms of God taking seriously, not our own sufferings, but those of God in the world—watching with [Jesus] in Gethsemane. . . . That is how one becomes a man."[9]

It is significant that one of the most important theologians of the twentieth century called for diminishing aspects of religious life that encourage institutional self-aggrandizement and preservation to focus on

---

5. Bonhoeffer, *Letters and Papers from Prison*, June 8, 1944, 168.

6. Bonhoeffer, *Letters and Papers from Prison*, April 30, 1944, 142.

7. Bonhoeffer, *Letters and Papers from Prison*, May 25, 1944, 164.

8. Bonhoeffer, *Letters and Papers from Prison*, July 16, 1944, 188.

9. Bonhoeffer, *Letters and Papers from Prison*, July 21, 1944, 193.

spiritual transformation that would result in transformed persons involved in service to the world. The juxtaposition of religion and spirituality is not new. Bonhoeffer's thoughts sound to me a lot like the principles found in the Twelve Steps of Alcoholics Anonymous. They sound like admitting that we are powerless (Step 1). They sound like in that experience of powerlessness coming to believe in a power greater than self that can bring not control, but sanity (Step 2). They sound like making "a decision to turn our will and our lives over to the care of God as we understood Him" (Step 3). Bonhoeffer sounds a lot like "praying only for knowledge of [God's] will for us and the strength to pursue it" (Step 11).

Alcoholics Anonymous Is Not Religious

I believe the spiritual program of recovery embodied in the Twelve Steps and in the Fellowship of A.A. can provide a model for religionless spirituality. It is important to recognize that for some, this spirituality will be linked to religion, while for others, it will not be; the spirituality exists independent of the degree or manner that any individual approaches or rejects religion. It is not averse to religion, nor is it dependent upon religion. What is consistent across members, regardless of their religious position, is that spiritual development through the spiritual principles and work of A.A. is the central focus for recovery. It is this central transformative spirituality that I believe can provide resources for those of us who are not part of the A.A. Fellowship.

A.A. clearly states that it is spiritual, not religious. Though A.A. has its roots in the Oxford Group, which was an interdenominational small-group religious movement, it quickly became a separate movement. The narrow focus in A.A. on alcoholism and its willingness to include any who desired to stop drinking meant some members were uncomfortable with religious language and the practices of the Oxford groups. From the beginning, the Fellowship of A.A. included the devoutly Christian, atheists and agnostics, and those concerned about turning people off with too much God talk. As the Big Book was being written, the content—especially the Steps—was hotly debated by members. Some thought it should be clearly Christian; others would accept the word "God" but were opposed to any other theological propositions; while others wanted to delete all reference to God and take a psychological approach. Compromises were finally developed: In Step 2, God was described as "a Power greater than ourselves."

In Steps 3 and 11, the term "God" was retained, but in the words "God as we understand Him." In Step 7, the words "on our knees" were removed. And perhaps most important, the Steps were described, not as essential doctrine, but as a "suggested program of recovery."[10] Thus with the intention of excluding theological doctrine (and the accompanying debates), the Big Book focused on what the founding members did to get and stay sober. It describes a plan of action; it avoids telling people what they should do or think or believe. As the Big Book says in introducing the Steps, "Here are the steps we took" (59). It is based on what worked, not on any theory or theology. As a result, today A.A. contains alcoholics of all faiths and of no traditional faith. While any member is at liberty to practice any religious doctrine, groups tend to share instead on the broad spiritual principles and practices that are uniform to all.

The spirituality contained in the Twelve Steps is the most effective means available for recovery. It is based on the experience of what works. A.A. is clear: the program is spiritual, not religious. It does not promulgate doctrine. It touches the hearts of those who suffer in hopelessness and despair.

I write to explore the question: In our secular society, where people profess they are spiritual but not religious, can the A.A. experience provide a pragmatic understanding of spirituality that heals, empowers, and restores relationships? The experience in the Fellowship of Alcoholics Anonymous provides a faith free of the mandates of religious doctrine, a spirituality that is pragmatic rather than theoretical, is transformational rather than analgesic, and is focused on concern for others rather than on doctrinal (or biblical) correctness. This spirituality can bring new life to the agnostic and the atheist, as well as to the traditionally religious. I seek to make clear that this pragmatic spiritual program of the Twelve Steps can provide support and transformation for all those who seek spiritual renewal today in our secular society.

---

10. Bill W., *Alcoholics Anonymous Comes of Age*, 162–67.

CHAPTER 2

Spiritual and Spirituality

A former inmate of a Nazi concentration camp was visiting a friend who had shared the ordeal with him.

"Have you forgiven the Nazis?" he asked his friend.

"Yes."

"Well, I haven't. I'm still consumed with hatred for them."

"In that case," said his friend gently, "they still have you in prison."[1]

THE SIMPLEST DEFINITION OF "spiritual" is anything that we cannot see or touch that affects our lives—things like love, resentment, hope, anger, acceptance, fear, peace, anxiety, and serenity. Spiritual realities are present for all human beings. When we become defensive because of criticism, that is a spiritual event. When we continue to hold a resentment against another, as in the story above, that is a spiritual dynamic that negatively impacts our lives. If we respond to an act of kindness with kindness in return, that is a spiritual event. A personal defeat may result in greater awareness of how others are hurt and beaten down, or in the resolve to avoid future defeat by never trying again, or in self-assessment and recognition of how others can help in the future, or any number of other responses. How one responds to defeat, kindness, hostility, support, or criticism depends on a very complex process we call "spirituality."

Spirituality is often associated with otherworldliness or the occult; sometimes with godliness or piety or purity. But it is much broader. It is the way we respond to events that are spiritual in nature. It is the way our

1. DeMello, *Heart of the Enlightened*, 107.

lives are organized with the result that certain responses and results become characteristic. One's spirituality may be conscious, but it also includes the unconscious. It may include intentional efforts, but it also includes unconsidered responses. Spirituality might be understood as experiences and principles that guide us in our actions and reactions to the world. Spiritual principles may provide direction when ideas or experiences are measured against them: "Is it honest?" "Is it unselfish?" "Is it an act of service?" "Do I gain from it?"

There is a tendency with many to dismiss "spiritual things" as ephemeral, unseen, and unimportant. "Sticks and stones may break my bones, but words can never hurt me." Never has any sentence been more untrue. It is usually spoken by someone who is trying to resist spiritually hurtful words. To believe it is to be blind to the reality of how hurtful and dispiriting words of enmity can be, or how helpful and joyful words of friendships can be. Spiritual realities have great power.

Spiritual realities are also legion; daily we are impacted by several powerful, invisible realities. Sunshine, a rainy day, a diagnosis of a serious illness, a good evaluation—or bad—by one's boss, all these events and many more may affect one's spirituality, one's sense of self, of security, of hopefulness. All communication is composed of an outward, visible act or event—snide remarks, fragrance, a hand, a smile, shunning, ignoring, a slap, a hug—and an inward, invisible aspect that the person interprets as hurtful, helpful, supportive, demeaning, anxiety-inducing, or satisfaction-producing. People respond largely on the basis of previous experience. Part of the difficulty of communication involves this invisible, spiritual component. A person may intend one thing, but the other person may perceive the act as something different. For example, when someone hugs another (visible act), the hug may be appreciated as warmth (invisible aspect) and a smile communicates the friendship, or it may be perceived as inappropriate (invisible aspect) and the person recognizes the need to be cautious toward a potentially abusive person. Past experience with the person or a similar experience with someone else will have an impact on the perception. A person's spirituality is the sum total, continually evolving, combination of responses to the multitude of spiritual events.

A person's spirituality, then, is built on three internal processes: 1) the way we perceive the world about us, 2) how we feel about that world, and 3) the choices we make—conscious and unconscious—in response to our perceptions and our sensations. These three processes are intertwined and mutually reinforcing:

Perception includes all the senses—sight, hearing, touch, taste, and kinesthesia. What is beautiful to one is not so to another; what tastes good to one may be bitter to another; a speaker may seem harsh to one person but inspiring to another. How one perceives reality depends on the person's experience, training, and abilities. Perception is not neutral:

> At noon in Times Square in New York, two men were making their way through the crowd, surrounded by the noise of the city. One was a native New Yorker; the other was a farmer from Kansas. Suddenly the farmer stopped. "Hold on," he said, "I hear a cricket."
>
> His friend replied, "Are you kidding? Even if there were a cricket around here, which seems most unlikely, you would never hear it above all this noise."
>
> The farmer remained quiet for a few moments, then walked over to a planter located a few paces away. He turned over several leaves and found the cricket. The New Yorker was flabbergasted.
>
> "What amazing hearing you have," he said.
>
> "No," the farmer replied, "it's a matter of what you've been conditioned to listen for. Let me show you." He pulled out a handful of coins from his pocket and let them drop on the sidewalk. Immediately several heads on the block turned to look.
>
> "You see," said the farmer, "you hear what you are accustomed to."[2]

Perception, then, is based in large part on likes, dislikes, fears, hopes, past experience, and the conditioning of the perceiver, who has developed these filters as a result of certain experiences and responses made over a lifetime.

Feelings that result from perception similarly influence perception and choices. What is the difference between laid-back and lazy? I would suggest the difference is with the one observing the laid-back/lazy person. If the observer likes the person, the person's actions will be filtered in a positive manner that characterizes him as relaxed, confident, laid-back; if the observer dislikes the person, the same actions will be seen as his wasting time, avoiding work, being lazy. The perceiver filters and interprets what is perceived on the basis of his or her own feelings and predispositions. Thus the damaging aspects of a friend's actions are diminished while those of someone who is disliked are stored as evidence why the person is unlikable.

2. Kurtz and Ketcham, *Experiencing Spirituality*, 111–12.

Choice may be the most subtle component in spiritual development. Most of our "choices" are unconscious reactions to an event or situation. They are automatic. Only if one is challenged is the choice consciously defended. It is far easier to blame others, blame the world, blame parents, make excuses, rationalize, justify, and twist facts than to take the time and energy for self-examination that can begin to identify patterns of behavior, resentment, and fear. As a result, many, perhaps most, people have little conceptualization of their personal participation in forming and maintaining their spiritual disposition.

In the 4th Step, the group member is challenged to make a "searching and fearless moral inventory" of themselves. In the 5th Step, they are to share it with God and another human being, admitting the "exact nature of" their wrongs. These are challenging Steps. With time, as one grows in self-acceptance, repeating them brings new insights and new abilities to see one's own participation in events that affect them. I have learned from these Steps that the only inventory I can take is my own. If I can let go of the fear, the insecurity, and the desire to blame, then I am able to see my part in what has happened and discover new choices I can make. I hope I practice this as much as I believe I do.

A person's spirituality, then, is the dynamic, complex, evolving combination of perception, feelings, and choices. It is more than seeing, more than feeling, more than choosing; it is the interplay and interconnection of all three. Perception is filtered to support a person's feelings and beliefs. Feelings and beliefs are reinforced by perception and choices. And choices are in response to these perceptions and feelings. This dynamic explains why once a person's understandings are formed, change is very difficult, even when the results of the person's spirituality make life unhappy.

Everyone has a spirituality, more or less considered, more or less intentionally nurtured. One person may be empathetic, having worked to develop strong listening skills and being able to understand the emotions another is feeling. One person may seek to avoid conflict whenever it emerges, agreeing by word or silence with the other's opinion and leaving when emotions become negative. The narcissist will interpret whatever happens as personal. Another may be a peacemaker and consciously work at finding the middle ground, assisting those in conflict to find understanding of the other and developing the tools of negotiation. These spiritualities formed by perception, feelings, and largely unconsidered choices serve as guides in our actions and reactions to the world.

Spirituality is a lot like health. We all have health; we may have good health or poor health, but it's something we can't avoid having. The same is true of spirituality: every human being is a spiritual being. The question is not whether we "have spirituality" but whether the spirituality we have is a negative one that leads to isolation and self-destruction or one that is more positive and life-giving.[3]

The desire to control illustrates the complexity of spirituality well. The parent whose teenager is drifting into alcohol and drug abuse wants more than anything to save the child from the pain and suffering that the parent can easily foresee. But the more the parent tries to control, the more the child resists. Anger, hostility, manipulation, and dishonesty from both parties act to escalate the conflict. Of course the parent is right; of course the teenager is headed for trouble; but the desire to control is defeating. We cannot control other people. We can give advice; we can encourage appropriate behavior; we can point out future probabilities; but we cannot control. The only person we can even seek to control is our self. The parent must develop a strong spirituality—a strong desire to control anger, a strong sense of self-esteem, a strong ability to accept the truth, a strong love for the child—to exercise tough love and, when necessary, to detach with love. The need to control is so great, but the teenager can only find recovery when he or she makes the choice to seek help. Controlling behavior damages the ability of the other to choose. Al-Anon provides a community that both supports and educates the parent, the spouse, or the friend as they seek to give choice to the other. Detaching means looking at oneself. Do I trust that there is a power greater than myself that seeks good for the other? Is my anxiety fueled by my own need to be seen as a normal, happy family? How do my fears, which we all have, make seeing the true situation difficult? Doesn't loving someone and caring about them mean keeping them safe when they have proven they cannot make good decisions? Dealing with the desire to control in the face of a real problem that cannot be controlled may force us to look at ourselves. The more we look, the more complex it becomes. We will have to deal with our own past, our own fears and anxieties, our own hopes, and above all, with our own powerlessness. One's spirituality and the ability to grow spiritually will be important factors in how one deals with such a situation. To grow spiritually is rarely comfortable. It requires

---

3. Dollard, quoted in Kurtz and Ketcham, *Spirituality of Imperfection*, 17.

deep self-reflection, changes in behavior, new ways of seeing, and making difficult choices. It usually requires help from others.

What, then, is spirituality? Found in the ordinary activities of life, spirituality represents how we put our experiences together—our painful times, our moments of joy, how others treat us, good and bad accidents that happen, love, neglect, abuse, sorrow, confusion—all responded to in accordance with our spirit. Spirituality describes the way we are, how we live.

> Someone asked a monk, "What is your life like as a monk?"
> The monk replied, "We walk, we fall down, someone helps us up. We walk some more, someone else falls down. We help them up. That's pretty much what we do."[4]

We all have a spirituality. Some seek to understand their way of coping and work to develop specific spiritual traits. Others may simply go through life, reacting to the immediate situation—angry when they do not get their way, happy when appreciated, sad at the death of a friend, anxious when confronted with any new situation—but without reflection on these spiritual events. Spirituality is a way of life; it is manifest throughout our interaction with ourselves and our world. It represents the way we perceive events and circumstances, how we feel about the world, and the choices we make. Spirituality is the evolving development of our understandings, of our acceptance of realities that surround us, and our commitment to tasks, persons, and things. It may be consciously developed or it may evolve without significant self-knowledge or reflection. Our spirituality has consequences.

Spirituality and the Sacred

We all are spiritual, but for many the understanding of spirituality is complicated by the concept of a transcendent God. Many of my atheist and agnostic friends prefer not even to use the word "spiritual" because they see it as a backdoor way of bringing God into the conversation. Others are comfortable talking about spirituality without believing in God. Among my more religious friends spirituality seems to mean primarily the religion they practice, including individual practices like corporate worship, prayer, study, and meditation. Spirituality means many different things to different people:

---

4. Kurtz and Ketcham, *Experiencing Spirituality*, 26.

There are these two guys sitting together in a bar in the remote Alaskan wilderness. One of the guys is religious, the other is an atheist, and the two are arguing about the existence of God with that special intensity that comes after about the fourth beer. And the atheist says: "Look, it's not like I don't have actual reasons for not believing in God. It's not like I haven't ever experimented with the whole God and prayer thing. Just last month I got caught away from the camp in that terrible blizzard, and I was totally lost and I couldn't see a thing, and it was 50 below, and so I tried it: I fell to my knees in the snow and cried out 'Oh, God, if there is a God, I'm lost in this blizzard, and I'm gonna die if you don't help me.'" And now, in the bar, the religious guy looks at the atheist all puzzled. "Well then you must believe now," he says, "After all, here you are, alive." The atheist just rolls his eyes. "No, man, all that was was a couple [Inuits] happened to come wandering by and showed me the way back to camp."[5]

There is a certain level of arrogance in both of these men. The nonreligious guy is totally certain in his dismissal of the possibility that the passing Inuits had anything to do with his prayer for help. But a similar level of arrogance in religious people, certain of their own interpretations, is equally repulsive. Religious dogmatists show a closed-mindedness that amounts to an imprisonment so total that they don't even know they are locked up. They are probably even more repulsive than atheists, at least to many of us.

There are these two young fish swimming along and they happen to meet an older fish swimming the other way, who nods at them and says "Morning, boys. How's the water?" And the two young fish swim on for a bit, and then eventually one of them looks over at the other and goes "What the hell is water?"[6]

We are seeking to develop a spirituality for our secular age. For many such a spirituality excludes dogmatism and even affiliation with a religious institution, but it does not automatically exclude belief in the Sacred. Because spirituality and relationship with the Transcendent are, for many, so totally connected, we must consider possibilities for a divine reality. What is the water that we as spiritual beings swim in? Are the powers that are greater than ourselves, that we cannot see or touch but which affect our lives, some sort of reality beyond ourselves? This question is beyond

---

5. Wallace, "This Is Water," para. 4.
6. Wallace, "This Is Water," para. 1.

knowing with certainty; therefore, to explore the idea that our world is somehow connected to an unseen divine reality requires humility.

How do members of A.A. find their higher power? Few come into the Fellowship with an existing relationship with God of any understanding. While each person's story is unique, there are several commonalities. They do not come to A.A. in order to grow spiritually or to find God; they come because their lives have become disastrously unmanageable as a result of alcohol and drug abuse. Out of the need to stop drinking and the inability to do this on their own, they find a power that empowers them to choose not to drink, at least for today. For many that power is identified as the God of their understanding. From the experience of powerlessness, the loving God who empowers is discovered.

The Big Book describes what we are calling "spiritual experience" in this way:

> Most of our experiences are what the psychologist William James calls the "educational variety" because they develop slowly over a period of time. Quite often friends of the newcomer are aware of the difference long before he is himself. He finally realizes that he has undergone a profound alteration in his reaction to life; that such a change could hardly have been brought about by himself alone. What often takes place in a few months could seldom have been accomplished by years of self-discipline. With few exceptions our members find that they have tapped an unsuspected inner resource which they presently identify with their own conception of a Power greater than themselves. (567–68)

It is common that many, having been empowered to achieve sobriety, seek to improve their conscious contact with God through prayer and meditation (Step 11). I do not think philosophical arguments for the existence of God play a large role with many in A.A. Personal experience is primary, but a secondary confirmation for many is reflecting on the coincidences in their lives. Many such stories are shared within A.A.; the following two come from Dr. Abraham J. Twerski, founder of the Gateway Rehabilitation Clinic where he has assisted more than 40,000 patients. He is a psychologist and a rabbi who found his calling working with alcoholics.

Dr. Twerski was traveling in his new car which he had driven less than 300 miles when the speedometer cable broke. He pulled into a filling station to get it repaired and saw two men standing in front of a car with the hood raised and steam rising from the motor. He recognized one of the men as a recent alumnus from the rehab center. The following are his words:

> "Hi, Doc!" he said. "Broken radiator hose; What's your problem?"
>
> "Broken speedometer cable," I said. "Brand-new car, too." I then proceeded to give him a tight hug. While the mechanic replaced my cable, I noticed that my friend was pacing to and fro like a caged animal. Eventually he came over and said, "Can you drop me off nearby, Doc?"
>
> When I told him I would, he told his friend to go on alone.
>
> Once we were in the car, I noticed my friend's forehead to be full of beads of perspiration, and he was visibly trembling.
>
> "You won't believe this, Doc," he said. "I've been clean for four months since I left Gateway. Today Frank came over and asked me if I wanted to go out with him. I was the one that turned Frank on to coke. My resistance broke down, and we were on our way to cop some coke when the radiator hose burst, and then you drove up."
>
> I parked the car and we talked a bit. I then suggested to my friend that I drop him off at a meeting. He is now seven years clean.[7]

The next story involves confusion resulting from two people who shared the same name. Seeking an appropriate A.A. contact for a patient who was in detoxification, Dr. Twerski called Ursula, who lived near the patient on the south side, to get a recommendation. Ursula was in her second year of recovery and had been attending A.A. She provided the name of a person to contact. When Dr. Twerski shared this with the unit nurse, a twelve-year veteran of A.A., she replied,

> "I hope you talked to Ursula about herself, because she has been drinking sporadically and has been slacking off in her meeting attendance."
>
> I was reluctant to believe that Ursula had relapsed, but when the nurse told me that she was Ursula's A.A. sponsor, I accepted the disappointing information.
>
> The following day when I called Ursula and thanked her for arranging the contact for my patient, I cautioned her: "I also want to tell you, Ursula, that you don't have to go all the way down in order to quit."
>
> "What do you mean?" she asked.

---

7. Twerski, *I'd Like to Call for Help*, 74–75.

"When you came in for treatment," I said, "you were in the pits. Although you have started drinking again, you don't have to get back to that terrible state. You can stop right where you are."

Ursula began crying. "How did you know?" she asked.

"How I know is totally irrelevant," I said, although I was a bit surprised that she did not realize that her sponsor and I are in frequent contact. "All I am asking of you is that you call your sponsor and get back to regular meetings!"

"Okay, I promise," she said. "But I can't understand how you found out."[8]

Later Dr. Twerski told the unit nurse about his conversation. They discovered that Dr. Twerski had called Ursula who lives on the south side when the nurse had recommended an Ursula who lives on the north side. Once more he called Ursula.

"I couldn't understand how you could have found out about my slip," she said. "After I left rehab, I was sober for over a year, then I drank for two days. I was okay for another few months and again I drank for only one day. This last week I again drank for only one day, but nobody knew about these slips. I hadn't even told my sponsor. It was so weird that you called me, because nobody knew."

While the universe is large beyond comprehension and the idea of a God who is concerned with what goes on with a single person on this one planet seems highly unlikely, Dr. Twerski reflects that events are more convincing than philosophy. "Obviously there can be such things as chance occurrences, but one reaches a point where ascribing things to chance or co-incidence requires a greater act of faith than belief in Divine intervention."[9]

Members of A.A. often refer to coincidences as miracles where God prefers to remain anonymous.

The experiences, the coincidences, and the sharing within the community that is Alcoholics Anonymous lead to recognition that we do not control our own lives and to the conviction by many that within this world there is a Benevolence that can be named "God." The Steps are careful not to describe this Transcendent Benevolence. Rather the individual seeks to build a pragmatic relationship that frees the person to be able to stay sober

8. Twerski, *I'd Like to Call for Help*, 72–74.
9. Twerski, *I'd Like to Call for Help*, 76.

today. We may not understand God, but by the grace of God we are happy, joyous, and free.

Within this discussion of spirituality, however, it seems important to go beyond this pragmatic understanding to briefly examine theological concepts. We do not see God, but for people of faith, who believe in God and practice some sort of spiritual discipline, God affects their lives deeply. When faith is central in their lives, it becomes a way of life. It forms how one perceives events and circumstances, how one feels about the world, and how one makes choices.

To have a relationship with the Transcendent, with a Power that is beyond perception and substantiation, may bring a strong sense of security and confidence to an individual. To believe that this world was created for a purpose, that our lives are not just cosmic accidents that have no reason for existing other than chance, means that the world is not hostile, that one can find purpose in his or her own life. To have a relationship with the Sacred may lead one to finding a place in life that is harmonious with others and with experience, to finding relationships and work that are mutually supportive, and to discovering a sense of serenity and peace despite hardships and disappointments.

To have a relationship with the Sacred is to discover that all of life is sacred. Yes, there is a great diversity of cultures, races, languages, sexual orientation, and ages—all are sacred. Every human being, created by God, is precious and honored and loved. Thus it is the norm within organized religion that there is a movement to empower members to work for justice and mercy. Divine Providence provides a spiritual foundation for such action.

> How long will it take? I come to say to you this afternoon however difficult the moment, however frustrating the hour, it will not be long, because truth pressed to earth will rise again. How long? Not long, because no lie can live forever. How long? Not long, because you will reap what you sow. How long? Not long, because the arm of the moral universe is long but it bends toward justice.[10]

To have a relationship with God, who is beyond knowing, is to grow in humility, in self-acceptance, in peace and serenity, in service to others in need, and in confidence in one's personal worth. We are not just an accident in a vast expanse of space; we are part of a beloved creation.

---

10. Martin Luther King Jr., in his address in Montgomery at the conclusion of the march from Selma, March 25, 1956 (King Jr., *Call to Conscience*, 131).

Many become intentional about their spiritual development through a religious community. In corporate worship we are affected by the music, especially in singing hymns. Such singing opens the heart to the Mystery that is found in the worshiping community. In corporate worship we may be engaged by the sermon to look at things in a new way or to be inspired to more vigorous service to those who are poor, discriminated against, or in prison. We are encouraged to do serious self-evaluation, expressing our sorrow for those things we believe we have done wrong and for those things we believe we should have done but did not do. Ritual provides a way of preserving one's relationship with the Divine Mystery without using emotional techniques to manipulate the believer. In personal reading, prayer, and meditation, we continue to seek insight, to express our concern for others, and to strengthen our conscious contact with God. At its best, religious experience will lead us in spiritual growth, healing our hurts and stimulating us to be more open to others, more open to change, and more able to accept the world as it is.

Many members of A.A. are also active in their churches. The Twelve Steps represent a spiritual program that will allow those who work the Steps to seek out and develop their spiritual values, priorities, and commitments. Many of these who are in recovery find that sacred space and religious communities support their spiritual development. And there are a few people like me who, even though they are not members of A.A., seek to use the Steps as their primary spiritual program. We find the rigor of this program, together with close friends in the recovering community, to be of great benefit in keeping us honest with ourselves and persistent in our practice of prayer and meditation.

Religion can be, should be, a primary source for healthy spiritual growth. Unfortunately, religion can also be a source for arrogant, negative spiritual development. How churches deal with the theological questions raised by faith may be a major factor in the health of their spirituality. Faith raises questions, and as Anselm, Archbishop of Canterbury(1093–1169). described theology, it is "faith seeking understanding."[11] We begin with faith and then humbly seek to understand the world, life, self, and spiritual mysteries. Human beings, however, seem to be uncomfortable with the ambiguity of "seeking answers"; we desire certainty. When churches decide that instead of seeking answers they have the answers, they are inclined to impose their understanding on their members and judge those whose

11. Williams, "Saint Anselm," sec. 2.1.

understandings differ. This claim to know the truth plays a central role in the churches developing a view of us versus them. At its worst, it has led to witch hunts, inquisitions, and persecutions; at its best, it leads to hypocrisy and arrogance—all in the name of the Sacred. Intolerance born of religious certainty is as old as the human desire for certainty and as destructive and ugly today as it has been in the past. To picture God through these lenses turns many today against religion. As noted earlier, many come to Alcoholics Anonymous having sought help from a church only to experience judgment—sometimes as subtle as the desire to help, sometimes as direct as condemnation of drunkenness. A spirituality seeking certainty easily becomes a spirituality of control and judgment that diminishes peoples' humanity. A spirituality of loving service heals, strengthens, liberates, motivates, reconciles, and in all ways enhances human life. Loving does not include theological certainty; it does involve commitment to others.

Former Archbishop of Canterbury Rowan Williams (2002–12) described the role of theology this way:

> If I have learned nothing else in fifty years, I have learned that a good theology is a theology oriented to healing of human wounds. And that witness to a new creation [must be] able to look with honesty at the failure, the guilt, and the pain of the world we're in, and yet to say that we are still called. We are still in the hands of a creator. We have a future."[12]

I firmly believe that a healthy spirituality nurtures human beings to be more accepting of themselves and more loving toward others. I have found such spirituality in both the recovering fellowship and in the church.

For many, perhaps most, believers, the word "God" refers to some sort of supernatural being, distinct from the universe—a supreme being who created the universe and who from time to time intervenes to keep the creation on track. This God also reigns as the supreme authority figure that tells us what we should believe and what is right and wrong. When combined with the idea that God is father to us all, this view provides, on the one hand, a relationship of intimacy, dependence, and protection, but on the other hand, may be interpreted as the authoritarian parent who criticizes, disciplines, and judges. Among my atheist and agnostic friends this supernatural parent theism is the view of God they find difficult to accept. I have many other friends who seem to speak in terms that sound like God is the super parent, but who recognize this is a far too simplistic

12. Williams, "Paddock Lectures at General Seminary," 12.

understanding. Rather this is a metaphor that enables their relationship with One who is far beyond our understanding.

There are other understandings and other experiences of God. Mystical experience forms the foundation of a very different way of thinking about God. I share the experience of my friend, the late Marcus Borg, a highly intellectual Jesus scholar, as he tells it in *Convictions: How I Learned What Matters Most.* At the time of this experience, he was in his early thirties, a time in his life when, as he describes it, his doubts about God were real and continued to deepen. Traditional theism simply made no sense in the light of scientific understandings. In part because of his doubts, he spent five years in graduate school studying the politics of Jesus. Then the following happened:

> I was driving through a sunlit rural Minnesota winter landscape alone in a nine-year-old MG two-seater roadster. The only sounds were the drone of the car and the wind through the thin canvas top. I had been on the road for about three hours when I entered a series of S-curves. The light suddenly changed. It became yellowy and golden, and it suffused everything I saw: the snow-covered fields to left and right, the trees bordering the fields, the yellow and black road signs, the highway itself. Everything glowed. Everything looked wondrous. I was amazed. I had never experienced anything like this before. . . .
>
> At the same time, I felt a falling away of the subject-object distinction of ordinary everyday consciousness—that "dome" of consciousness in which we experience ourselves as "in here" and the world as "out there." I became aware not just intellectually but experientially of the connectedness of everything. I "saw" the connectedness, experienced it. My sense of being "in here" while the world was "out there" momentarily disappeared.
>
> That experience lasted for maybe a minute and then faded. But it had been the richest minute of my life.[13]

He writes that for the next two years he experienced more moments like this one. And then one more twenty years later. At the time he was not aware of mysticism in Christianity or any other religions. Soon after these experiences he accepted a teaching appointment through which he became familiar with William James's *Varieties of Religious Experience.* Only then did he realize what had happened was a mystical experience.[14]

13. Borg, *Convictions,* 36.
14. Borg, *Convictions,* 36–37.

James, in his classic book, describes mystical experiences, concluding that their two primary features are "illumination" and "union." Illumination involves light and radiance, but includes a new way of seeing, enlightenment. Union refers to the experience of connectedness and the disappearance or softening of the distinction between self and the world. In addition, James names four other common features:

Ineffability: The experiences are difficult, even impossible, to express in words.

Transiency: They are usually brief; they come and go.

Passivity: One cannot make them happen through personal effort.

Noetic quality: They include a vivid sense of knowing—a nonverbal, nonlinguistic way of knowing marked by a strong sense of seeing more clearly.[15]

As Dr. Borg notes,

> The question of God's existence is no longer about whether there is another being in addition to the universe. Rather the question becomes . . . What is reality? Is it simply the space-time world of matter and energy as disclosed by ordinary sense perception and contemporary science? Or is it suffused by a "more," a radiant and glorious more? A theology that takes mystical experiences seriously leads to a very different understanding of the referent of the word "God." The word no longer refers to a being separate from the universe, but to a reality, a "more," a radiant and luminous presence that permeates everything that is.[16]

When in the Acts of the Apostles Luke records Paul as referring to God as "[the one in whom] we live and move and have our being (Acts 17:28) is he describing the mystic's experience of God?

If God is love, does this mean we are surrounded on every side by love in good times and difficult times if only we have eyes to see and ears to hear?

Is this water, the water in which we live and move and have our being?

To conclude, when we speak of spirituality, we must first recognize that human beings are spiritual; we all have a spirituality and react/respond to spiritual forces that surround us. And second, we recognize that the

---

15. James, as summarized in Borg, Convictions, 38–39.
16. Borg, Convictions, 44–45.

invisible reality often referred to as God comes with an infinite number of possible understandings, and that those who believe in God use language that is metaphorical, not descriptive. What I like about Twelve-Step spirituality is that it focuses on the first—how we can mature spiritually—without getting caught in the difficulties and disagreements on the nature of God.

CHAPTER 3

Twelve-Step Spirituality

WITHOUT QUESTION THE TWELVE Steps lay out a spiritual program, but it is a spirituality based on experience, not doctrine. The Steps do not promulgate a theology. The basic text of A.A. is entitled *Alcoholics Anonymous*, after the movement from which it was authored. It is fondly referred to as the Big Book. It states: "The spiritual life is not a theory. *We have to live it*" (83; italics original). Central in the spirituality of A.A. is mystery, not doctrine—mystery at the miracle of lives changed by following these simple principles.

A very powerful spiritual transformation takes place as a function of working these Steps that are the core teaching in *Alcoholics Anonymous*. Most members will tell you that when they came to A.A. they were seeking relief from compulsive, destructive consumption of alcohol; they were not in pursuit of a spiritual experience. Yet, the spiritual reorganization occurs, not because it is sought, but as a function of spiritual action through the Steps. The relief they seek is a by-product of the spiritual transformation that occurs as a result of working through the Twelve Steps. This program is able to touch the hearts of those who suffer hopelessness and despair.

Twelve-Step spirituality is far more than just the Twelve Steps. The spirituality of Alcoholics Anonymous includes the Steps; it also includes the Twelve Traditions, the Big Book, the Preamble, the use of sponsors, printed sayings that are common to members, wisdom from old-timers, the reflected wisdom of group members, other books like *Twelve Steps and Twelve Traditions*, the *Grapevine* magazine, and above all, stories.[1] How-

1. The Preamble, the Twelve Steps, and the Twelve Traditions are found in Appendix A.

ever, the Twelve Steps are the core spiritual guides that are the heart of the A.A. program.

This spiritual approach has proved so successful that many other programs have adopted the core Twelve Steps as it relates to a specific problem, including Al-Anon, Narcotics Anonymous, Gamblers Anonymous, Overeaters Anonymous, and more than one hundred and fifty other groups. We also learn from these fellowships.

Finally, when I speak of Twelve-Step spirituality, I am sharing my personal experience. There are many who may have different understandings of the spirituality they find in the Fellowship of Alcoholics Anonymous.

This rich diversity of views comes largely because A.A. offers not a theory, not a hypothesis, not doctrine, not theology, not a pious hope, not wistful or wishful thinking, but a record of how alcoholics achieved sobriety. In "How It Works," the fifth chapter in the Big Book, there is no examination of the causes of alcoholism, no theory about a cure. The format is simple: "This is what we did," a sharing of experience, drinking and sobriety. Experience is the first principle. The Big Book contains stories by those who found sobriety by following the Steps. A.A. spirituality is built on the experience of what works. There is considerable latitude to be found in the application of the principles and actions associated with the Steps. This leads to a variety of understandings. What works for one person is not necessarily what works for another. Still there is an overall coherent consistency within A.A. that provides a unity of spirit within the diversity of experience.

Twelve-Step spirituality is pragmatic, focusing on what works; it is centered in a community; it is inclusive, welcoming all who desire to stop drinking; it seeks to be rigorously honest even when that honesty involves questioning faith; it centers upon service to the still-suffering alcoholic; and it is transformational. Participants move from despair to hope, from self-focused resentment to concern for others, and from angry efforts seeking control to gratitude for gifts received. It can provide support and insight for all.

Some fundamental elements of Twelve-Step spirituality are described in what follows. While others might approach this differently, I hope these elements represent the overall consistency found in Twelve-Step spirituality.

Spiritual Transformation

The heart of the program is spiritual transformation. Because alcoholism is a physical, mental, and spiritual disease, in addition to physical healing a spiritual healing is also needed. No one freely chooses to be an alcoholic. No one gets up in the morning and says, "I think today would be a good day to see if I can get a DWI." People develop the disease over a period of time, and when the person has become addicted, two particular characteristics dominate the person.

Having become dependent on the drug, experiencing anxiety, depression, and withdrawal if unable to obtain a drink, most alcoholics become compulsively preoccupied to make certain it will be available. Elaborate schemes of hiding bottles, stealing money for drinks, and otherwise assuring the availability of the drug are typically present. We are coming to understand that the brain has been reprogrammed so the alcoholic or addict feels substantial anxiety or desperation if they cannot get a drink. When the alcoholic says, "If I do not get a drink, I will die" that is not hyperbole; that is what they are feeling and believing.

The other characteristic is a loss of control after one drink. The first drink inevitably leads to another and another *ad infinitum*. The consequences of this repeated behavior are destructive to the drinker and to those who are close to him or her. To the nonalcoholic this behavior seems baffling; to alcoholics the drug is a power they become unable to control. Distortions in thinking, expectations, and desires interfere with any capacity for a clear review of circumstances. As the first Step says, alcoholics are powerless over alcohol and their lives have become unmanageable. Contemporary brain research is beginning to cast light on how thinking is affected by addiction. In fact alcoholics are unable to make the choices they desire to make and make choices that are ultimately self-destructive.

A.A. spirituality is about transformation from powerlessness to becoming able to make desired choices. The domination by compulsion and loss of control mean the alcoholic is unable, by his or her own will power, to control drinking or the consequences of drinking. Restoration of the ability to choose represents a spiritual transformation, a personality change sufficient to bring about recovery. By definition it is dependent upon a power outside the individual, since of their own accord alcoholics are unable to make these choices. Individuals choose how to understand this power for themselves, with an amazing latitude for how it is defined as long as it is understood as stronger than the individual alone. Almost any conceptualization is allowed—some are rooted in traditional theology, but other concepts acceptable to the seeker are allowed. Some may begin by considering an A.A. group as this power, as together this group is thought to have more ability than the alcoholic alone. Recognizing the diverse nature of individual spiritual experience, the Steps avoid doctrinal or theoretical definitions of this power to restore sanity and choice by using the terms "Higher Power" or "God of one's understanding."

This "Higher Power" is often thought of as being beyond the individual. It represents a power not previously known that gives the alcoholic the ability to choose. This transformation and this Power are best understood as a spiritual event. Dr. Harry Tiebout, the first psychiatrist to support A.A. and an early friend of Bill W., said it this way, "A religious or spiritual experience is the act of giving up reliance on one's own omnipotence."[2]

There are many kinds of spiritual experiences. Some are like the conversions of the great religious leaders of the past; others seem purely psychological. Some are sudden or instantaneous; others are a gradual learning process. But all of them, whatever form they take, have one effect: they make a person capable of doing something she or he could not do before. As Bill W. puts it, "When a man or a woman has a spiritual awakening, the most important meaning of it is that he has now become able to do, feel, and believe that which he could not do before on his unaided strength and resources alone."[3] Bill found confirmation of this understanding in William James's book *Varieties of Religious Experience*. Summarizing James, Bill wrote, "Not only . . . could spiritual experiences make people saner, they could transform men and women so that they could do, feel, and believe what had hitherto been impossible to them. It mattered little whether these awakenings were sudden or gradual; their variety could be almost infinite."[4] The test of the validity of the Steps, the Twelve Traditions, the group sharing, sponsorship, and the other tools used in A.A. is not some intellectual theory or a belief system; the test of the validity of A.A. spirituality is the pragmatic recognition that it works. And there are millions whose lives testify to this reality.

Spiritual transformation implies a change of consciousness: a new set of eyes and ears to perceive the world, a new set of behaviors that slowly

2. Bill W., *Language of the Heart*, 99.

3. Bill W., *Twelve Steps and Twelve Traditions*, 106.

4. Bill W., *Language of the Heart*, 197.

become natural, a new openness to others, and a new sense of gratitude that brings with it an obligation to serve those who still suffer.

For many in the beginning, the Higher Power is simply a voice from outside that allows the person to begin the journey toward sobriety and freedom. Later the person may discover an inner resource that leads to the personality change that provides the strength to overcome addiction. With this spiritual growth, members often express the sense that letting a Higher Power be in charge has resulted in their being more truly themselves. This rebirth of a more authentic self, free from addiction, free from the bondage of self, and becoming free from shame, guilt, hopelessness, and loneliness—this rebirth is a miracle, beyond simple explanations. Some may see this transformation as a simple rearrangement—a function of different thinking, feeling, interpretation, and action. Others may see a spiritual miracle is the result of divine grace—a gift unearned, undeserved, and freely bestowed by God.

Meetings

The most obvious aspect of Twelve-Step spirituality is meetings. The power of meetings is discussed more fully in chapter 6, but we cannot begin to consider A.A. spirituality without talking about meetings. Meetings are characteristic not only of A.A. but also of N.A. (Narcotics Anonymous), Al-Anon, and all the other more than 150 programs based on the Steps.

When the Big Book was first published, surprisingly, regular group meetings were not seen as part of the program. Instead, there was much more focus on the use of the book, application of the Steps, and Twelfth-Step calls, which were efforts to share about A.A. with prospective members in hospitals and institutions. However, even in the beginning, small groups were meeting. In the very beginning, after co-founders Bill Wilson and Dr. Bob Smith met, they continued for awhile to meet with groups that were part of the Christian, nondenominational Oxford Groups. The religious character of the Oxford Groups was in tension with Bill and Bob's focus on reaching out to alcoholics, regardless of their faith or denomination. As a result, the new groups separated from the Oxford Groups. The Big Book was published in 1939. In 1941, Jack Anderson wrote a compelling article in the *Saturday Evening Post* that led to an explosion of interest in Alcoholics Anonymous and requests for help. Membership grew from 2,000 to 8,000! Groups sprang up all over the country, using only the Big

Book as a guide. The power of the groups was evident in the natural and often unprompted manner with which they sprung forth.

With the expansion of groups came a plethora of problems. Among the most important issues was who could be members. In the beginning, groups were very concerned and developed all sorts of rules to restrict membership. There was concern about what to do with slips; there was concern about criminals; concern about social status, race, gender, age—all sorts of concerns. An early event occurred when a group contacted Bill W. about two African Americans who wanted to attend. There was much discussion back and forth. Would welcoming a Negro damage the fledgling young program? Finally they asked, "Is he a drunk? Does he want to get sober?"[5] When the response came back in the positive, the issue was settled; he was welcome.

The felt need for rules is not surprising. The group and the program of Alcoholics Anonymous had literally saved lives. What saved one person's life would naturally be seen as the right way. Rules seemed to preserve this "right way." As each group developed its structure and rules, the number of rules expanded. As Bill W. expressed later, there were so many rules about membership in the different groups that if they were all enforced, no one would be able to join. The issue was initially settled when the Big Book was published. In the foreword was written, "The only requirement for membership is an honest desire to stop drinking."[6] Even this proved to be too restrictive. As the Twelve Traditions were developed, the word "honest" was dropped. Who could determine if the person's desire to stop drinking was "honest"? A person is a member if he or she says so. It is as simple as that.

Thus a fundamental character of the A.A. groups was established. They are to be open to all who are powerless to control their addiction and have a desire to stop drinking. This radically inclusive quality has resulted in two dynamics: First, the membership of A.A. is amazingly diverse. Male, female, old, young, Black, Hispanic, White, well educated, poorly educated, hopeless street drunks, still functioning alcoholics, Catholic, Protestant, Jew, Hindu, agnostic, atheist, gay, straight, American, European, Asian, English speaking, non-English speaking—by 1945 all of these categories and more were found among the members. And all were discovering that if they worked the Steps, they could become free from the cunning, baffling, powerful disease of alcoholism. And second, despite this diversity there is a

---

5. *A.A. for the Black African American Alcoholic*, 6.

6. Bill W., *Alcoholics Anonymous Comes of Age*, 102.

strong sense of unity within the Fellowship of A.A., as there is an underlying commonality found in their personal history of alcoholism and their recovery through following this simple program.

Shortly after *Alcoholics Anonymous* was published, as the number of groups expanded without a common prescription for organization or function, a recently sober promoter developed an idea for how to move the organization forward. His plan included three separate corporations to spread the message. He would develop a single large building with a club, a meeting area, a clinic, and a loan office. He submitted his blueprint, outlined in sixty-one rules, regulations, and by-laws to A.A.'s New York headquarters requesting a "super charter." Bill responded with his usual format: experience tells us that such grandiose plans have failed elsewhere before, but your group has the right to ignore this warning. It did and the "thump of colliding egos could be heard and felt for miles" as the project crashed. In time, the furor quieted, and the chastened promoter wrote New York again. His letter admitted that headquarters was right, and he enclosed a card he had already mailed to every A.A. group in the United States. On the front of the card was printed "Group [the location]—Alcoholics Anonymous: Rule No. 62." When the card was opened a single sentence met the eye: "Don't take yourself too damned seriously."[7] The laughter one finds in every A.A. group testifies to how Rule 62 has become a part of group life.

Faced with the question of how A.A. and the groups should be organized—more control or minimal organized structure—Bill W. consistently clung to his commitment that there was to be no central authority and therefore only minimal organizational structure. Just as the Twelve Steps were written for the individual alcoholic as a path to recovery, now ideas for the well-being of groups were needed. From the experience of the groups a set of twelve traditions began to emerge. Bill's commitment to minimal organization is reflected in them. For the groups there is only one authority, "a loving God as He may express Himself in our group conscience. Our leaders are but trusted servants; they do not govern" (Tradition 2). The groups are "autonomous except in matters affecting other groups or A.A. as a whole" (Tradition 4).

This was not without criticism. Dr. Harry Tiebout saw in this renunciation of authority an abdication of responsibility and voiced his concern emphatically. Bill's reply was that "great suffering and great love are A.A.'s disciplinarians; we need no others." The groups could be autonomous

7. Bill W., *Alcoholics Anonymous Comes of Age*, 103–4.

because, guided by a loving God as known through the group conscience, they provided a freeing, loving, healing community. If one deviated from the group norms enough, the penalty for drunkenness is insanity or death. "We can simply leave the job [of governance] to John Barleycorn."[8]

The explosion of membership after the publication of the Jack Allen *Saturday Evening Post* article in 1941 resulted in an explosion of groups. The old method of personal visits from existing groups to new groups soon proved inadequate. The increase in correspondence with Bill placed major stress on the small central office. There was a need for guidance for the groups, which today are clearly the heart of the program. The development of the Twelve Traditions, first published in 1946 in the *Grapevine*, were to meet the concerns from the groups. As Bill said, "The Twelve Traditions are to group survival and harmony what A.A.'s Twelve Steps are to each member's sobriety and peace of mind."[9] Or as I have heard many members say, "The Steps saved me from killing myself; the Traditions save us from killing each other."

Like the Twelve Steps, the Twelve Traditions are based on experience. The challenge was how to share the accumulating wisdom of experience from the groups without establishing a central authority which might stifle further experience and greater wisdom. The solution was based on the sharing of challenges and questions through correspondence. By 1945, with membership having grown to over 15,000, many of the questions had become repetitive and the group experiences both good and disastrous had evolved into a set of principles that might be codified into the Twelve Traditions. In many ways they represent what not to do based on the problems and conflicts the groups experienced.

Bill's leadership in developing the Traditions appears to have been based on two spiritual principles derived from his own experience and the experience shared from the groups. The first of these was a strong sense of limitation. Sober alcoholics are made whole by their acceptance of their limitations. They are unable to achieve sobriety alone; they need a power greater then themselves to be made free. They may not even resolve to remain sober more than one day. The alcoholic is not God; the alcoholic is a limited human being. In a similar way, A.A. as a fellowship is also limited. A.A. is human, not God. It exists only to serve sobriety. As an alcoholic must find a Higher Power to find recovery, so too the groups must depend

8. Kurtz, *Not-God*, 107–8.

9. Bill W., *Alcoholics Anonymous Comes of Age*, 96.

not on organizational structure but on the will of a loving God as expressed in the group conscience.

The other principle—the avoidance of grandiosity—mirrors the first. Grandiosity is a constant temptation that invites the alcoholic to delude him or herself that drinking moderately is an option. Having achieved sobriety, former drunks could convince themselves that they had the answers to all of life's problems, that they should be paid as professional counselors, that with appropriate publicity they could save thousands more drunks. Experience had taught how dangerous such thinking was both for the individual and also for the Fellowship of Alcoholics Anonymous.

The Traditions were developed to provide guidelines for relationships: relations of the individual to the A.A. group, the relations of A.A. to the group, and the place of Alcoholics Anonymous to society. The group and its members were to avoid problems of money, property, and prestige in order to focus on the mission of carrying the message of hope to those who still suffer from this disease.

Thus the groups became central and the authority for the group actions lies with those who attend. Why the groups became central seems clear when we understand that alcoholism is a disease of isolation. A friend tells me the only thing she remembers from her first meeting is that a member told her, "You will never again have to face your problems alone." This isolation, plus the alcoholic's capacity for denial and self-deception, means the alcoholic cannot recover alone. James Nelson describes how important the group continues to be in recovery.

> I need reminders from others when I take inventory of my life. I need to unburden myself to others, tell my story, and listen carefully to others' stories. I need the relief that someone else knows what it's like. I need to extend my help to others, not only for their sakes, but also to reinforce my own sobriety. In short, I need a community with whom I can share experience, strength, and hope.[10]

Rigorous Honesty

In A.A. spirituality there is a focus on honesty as essential to transformation and recovery. Those who are "incapable of grasping and developing a

---

10. Nelson, *Thirst*, 183.

manner of living which demands rigorous honesty" will be unable to find recovery. However, even those "who suffer from grave emotional and mental disorders, [may] recover if they have the capacity to be honest" (85). Rigorous honesty is one of the most difficult tasks any human being can undertake. For alcoholics who have been denying they are dependent on the drug, honestly admitting they are addicted and need help is the difference between life and death.

I remember a visit I made to a parishioner who had two beautiful young daughters and whose husband had multiple arrests related to his drinking. He was a carpenter, but their home needed a variety of repairs he could easily do. Though he worked regularly, they were clearly struggling financially. His father had died as a result of his alcoholism. I made the call to encourage her to begin attending Al-Anon. Ours was a warm relationship, but this visit soon turned cool. She said her husband had been unlucky in being arrested. She insisted that they were doing well. She did not believe there was any need for help for her or for her husband. She seemed unable to see what seemed obvious to many of those who loved and cared for that family.

I find myself baffled as to how a person can go through a gastrointestinal illness, a warning from an employer regarding job performance, pleading and threatening from a spouse, and arrests for DWI, and still not see the obvious: alcohol is a problem, and if I cannot stop drinking on my own, I need help. It is truly baffling, but I also recognize that such denial of the obvious is only a somewhat exaggerated form of the way all of us develop spiritually. Our perceptions are filtered by our hopes, our fears, our conditioning, and our self-assessment. I think of myself as a good driver. Therefore, I ignore the times my tires hit the rumble strip; I ignore when I am sleepy and keep on driving; I ignore that I ignore the speed limit; I ignore my age and the data on elderly drivers. As long as I am not in an accident where I am at fault, I think of myself as a good driver. Rigorous honesty dampens a lot more than just drinking. Perceiving reality as it is and not as I want it to be is a skill that takes great effort and assistance; it does not come naturally.

Denial is a normal part of what human beings do in order to cope with discouraging realities in life. Denial is not rationalization or justification; it is firmly believing something that is not true about oneself or about another who is an important part of one's life. Behind rationalization and justification is the recognition of the facts of what actually happened. As a result there is suspicion by the person that he or she may not be correct in dismissing the event. Denial is much stronger than rationalization because the person firmly believes he or she is correct. What is so baffling in dealing with an active alcoholic or drug addict is how can they continue to deny when the evidence continues to accumulate and the consequences are insanity or death. Acceptance of reality is essential to recovery—in addiction and in all of life. Rigorous honesty is modeled strongly in sharing in A.A. meetings and is the cornerstone of a relationship with a sponsor, who is a sober member who serves to guide another member, usually with less time sober, through the Steps.

An important piece of wisdom gained from the early days of A.A. is that sharing experiences is helpful, while pointing out the difficulties and disasters is not. The first drunk Bill W. and Dr. Bob sought to assist by sharing their personal stories was Bill D. (often referred to as A.A. #3). They were successful because their stories lit a spark of hope within Bill D. As he tells his story, his wife "had been talking to a couple of fellows about drinking. I resented this very much, until she informed me that they were a couple of drunks just as I was. That wasn't so bad, to tell it to another drunk." She told me they had a plan and it included sharing the plan with another drunk and that would help them stay sober. "All the other people who had talked to me wanted to help *me*, and my pride prevented me from listening to them and caused only resentment on my part, but I felt as if I would be a real stinker if I did not listen to a couple of fellows for a short time, if that would cure *them*." As Bill W. relates the story, when he and Dr. Bob returned a second day, they "found Bill with his wife Henrietta. Eagerly he pointed to [them] saying, 'These are the fellows I told you about; they are the ones who understand'" (188–89; italics original). Rigorous honesty is one of the most fundamental elements embedded in the Twelve Steps, in its admission of powerlessness over alcohol, in its searching and fearless moral inventory, and in its seeking spiritual development. Such honesty is essential when one shares personal experience, and this sharing brings the possibility of an identification that opens the door of hope. Rigorous honesty is also powerfully modeled in the context of the A.A. group and in the sponsor relationship.

Honesty provides the opportunity for humility. Bill W. and Dr. Bob connected with Bill D. because they were totally honest, sharing in great detail the disaster that had been their lives. This combination of humility and honesty, combined with the fact that they were now sober, allowed the seed of hope to begin to take root. Bill D. was able to hear their stories because there was no judgment; they had lived what he was living. Straightforward, honest, nonjudgmental telling connected and led to a breakthrough, overcoming his denial. Of course Bill D. needed to continue to seek rigorous honesty if he was to have any hope of continuing recovery and not returning to his well-practiced denial and lies. This peer-to-peer dynamic explains why I, as one who is not an alcoholic and has not lived through what alcoholics go through, cannot make Twelfth-Step calls. No matter how humble and honest I seek to be, I have not experienced what they are going through; I will come across as some one who wants to help—always an implied judgment.

What I experienced in my little group of recovering alcoholics that met every Tuesday afternoon was this spirit of honesty. There was one primary concern: that we be honest about our lives, our doubts, our experiences, and our insights. For the first time in my life as a religious leader, no one cared what I had done or what I was thinking or whether the congregation was growing. They cared only that I be as honest as possible with myself and to them about my experience. No one had to say out loud that was our standard; we all knew. That spirit was freeing and transforming.

After I left Louisville, I sought to set up a support group with other clergy. We had some wonderful conversations and some good sharing about our work, but that criterion of rigorous honesty was not present; the personal sharing was less thorough. I learned that when I included a recovering alcoholic who was active in A.A., the level of honest sharing changed dramatically. Because of their experience they have a remarkable BS detector. For the remainder of my ministry I have always included someone from the A.A. Fellowship in my support groups.

Rigorous honesty is difficult, often painful, and challenging, but it is also freeing, leading to life-giving self-acceptance. It is essential to recovery, as it allows for self-examination, responsibility, and spiritual growth. Honesty engenders humility, as we see who we are and the world as it is. Honesty rightsizes us to the world and to those around us.

Surrender and Humility

I believe the fundamental spiritual experience in A.A. is the movement from being self-directed—I can control my drinking, I am strong, I need to control you—to being directed by a power greater than self. "First of all,"

Bill says, "we had to quit playing God. It didn't work" (62). It is a movement toward recognition that we are not God, we cannot control our life or the lives of others, and that seeking such control actually makes life unmanageable. Be assured, this fundamental understanding of what is, of who we are, is humility. Importantly, it is not humiliation. Though the freshly sober person may have a myriad of issues and episodes that will require attention and accounting for, the principle that begins to emerge with a constant state of honesty and searching is humility. A.A., then, is a movement toward letting go of all that baggage and accepting that we must find a new way of living that is directed by a Higher Power, a new way of living that includes reaching out to others who still suffer from addiction.

Some in A.A. summarize that the Twelve Steps are an ego-deflating process, where one faces one's alcoholism, surrenders to the fact that alone they have insufficient power to overcome the compulsion to drink, seeks to identify and make amends for past harms, and then continues to behave in a manner leading to awareness, responsibility, and community. This is infused throughout the Twelve-Step process.

"Surrender" is a word that is often misunderstood. People hear a negative tone in the concept. For some people, like those in the military, surrender is a particularly difficult word. Surrender for the soldier is unacceptable. Similarly for most of us, it sounds like resignation, defeat, and despair. In this examination of Twelve-Step spirituality, we must be clear that surrender is a positive act; it is the opposite of resignation. Resignation means to cease to struggle because one is defeated; resignation is to give up and accept defeat, knowing it will lead to insanity, jail, and death. Surrender is a positive act. First, it means accepting the world as it is and not trying to create life according to one's own terms. Part of that acceptance is the reality that one is alcoholic, that things are as they are. Surrender involves abandoning the strategic use of control to achieve one's goals and accepting that with help one can be relieved of the obsession to drink. Surrender of self is necessary to become part of the greater whole—the local meeting, the worldwide Fellowship, the world. Surrender means we are no longer alone or isolated. Surrender is the beginning of change, the embracing of a new way that leads to a new life. Sometimes resignation and surrender look alike, but the difference between them is the difference between death and life.

Surrender, turning one's "will and life over to the care of God as we understood Him," (Step 3) means accepting some radically new ways of living. It includes open-mindedness, openness to a different point of view, and willingness to take advice and try some new ways of doing things. Surrender means letting go of "my way or the highway," and accepting guidance from the experience of sober members of A.A. and getting a sponsor who will be a companion in recovery. Surrender means accepting those things we cannot change—our history, our addiction, our fears, our shame, our desire for control—and changing those things that we can while seeking wisdom from God and from others. Surrender is the first step in a process of spiritual growth that will result in transformation, from addiction to sobriety, from powerlessness to becoming able to make desired choices.

Resentment, Bondage to Self

The Big Book says that "resentment is the 'number one' offender. It destroys more alcoholics than anything else" (64). Nonalcoholics find this statement startling. They think it is alcohol that destroys the alcoholic. They do not understand the importance of spiritual health for recovery. The Big Book goes on to explain, "From [resentments] stem all forms of spiritual disease." To straighten out physically and mentally, one must overcome such spiritual maladies.

Resentment is a primary symptom of the bondage to self that is at the heart of not only the alcoholic but at the heart of our human problem. Resentment focuses us on ourselves as having been offended by others. It is less a feeling and more a way of seeing. I have been injured; they are to blame; I am a victim. As long as we wallow in self-pity and focus on "poor me," we will never grow. We are like a man stuck in a cesspool, when someone offers a rope to allow him to climb out, he calls back, "No, teach me to swim without making waves." We know there are those who have been destroyed because they were so wrapped up in their system of blame, especially in how they had been wronged.

The solution to resentment and to the bondage of self is to let go by turning our will and our lives over to the God of our understanding (Step 3), which is practiced again and again as needed. Turning our will and lives over to God involves seeing the world in a whole new way. We must let go of the past, which we cannot change. We must let go of seeking to control others and outcomes of events. We must let go of evaluating results, which is a focus on self—what a successful person I am, or what a failure I am. The Steps provide tools to help us let go. Make a fearless moral inventory, share it with God and another person, make amends to those harmed, and pray for the removal of "every single defect of character which stands in the way of my usefulness to [God] and [other human beings]" (76). We have to let go of trying to understand everything; let go of the desire to have all the right answers; let go of the need to be right, let go of the desire to be the savior. We must learn to accept the world as it is, not as we wish it were and learn to accept ourselves as we are and not as we pretend to be. We can appreciate how working the Steps will stifle resentment, fear, and self-centeredness, allowing the person to return to a surrendered, humble, open state.

If there is anything I have learned from A.A. it is that the only inventory I can take is my own. When I begin to own my responsibility for some of what happens to me, when I have a group where I can share honestly what has happened, including my own faults, and when the group, knowing its own shortcomings, kindly admonishes me to stop feeling sorry for myself, when there is a spirit of acceptance and humor and recognition that all of us fall short of perfection, then I discover that I have begun to accept myself, to accept others, to let go of my resentments, and to live in this world as it is, not as I would try to create it.

Service

The Twelfth Step asks members to carry the message to the still-suffering alcoholic. It is another significant push toward moving away from self and toward community and usefulness. This Step contains the focus on service that is essential to Twelve-Step spirituality. The Big Book speaks of the "bondage of self." When one is drinking alcoholically, the focus is totally on self. There is guilt because of the consequences of bad behavior. There is shame in the inability to control one's drinking. There is fear of others' judgments, of others' anger, of others' disdain. There is the constant effort to control those who would prevent the acquisition of alcohol and who might destabilize the delicate balance the alcoholic seeks to preserve. And there are resentments against all those who interfere. The focus is totally on self, and alcoholics are unable to be free from this focus. They must control their drinking, be strong, and control those who would prevent their drinking. By moving through the Steps and the process of reckoning with one's past, and developing a community and what some would consider an awareness of God or a power greater than themselves around them, the alcoholic becomes much less interested in self and is able to engage in the greater world. Becoming of service by helping others, being responsible to a "home group" and their A.A. community, and also contributing to non-A.A. endeavors, the now-sober alcoholic becomes enriched and rewarded, sustained in purpose and community.

And as one begins to be freed from the bondage of self, as one begins to see the world as it is, our eyes are opened to see both the love that surrounds us on every side and the pain and sorrow that surround us as well. When alcoholics see another still suffering from this disease, knowing one of the ways to be free from the focus on self is to focus on another, they reach out with a "Twelfth-Step call" to share their story with the hope that the other may find hope. However, knowing they are not the savior, they offer their assistance and leave the results in God's and the drinker's hands. Such action is freeing for both the one in recovery and the one still imprisoned by the disease.

When one works the Steps, one of the results is a life devoted to service. In the words of a couple of members:

> When I talk with a newcomer to A.A., my past looks me straight in the face. I see the pain in those hopeful eyes. I extend my hand, and then the miracle happens: I become healed. My problems vanish as I reach out to this trembling soul.

> While practicing service to others, if my successes give rise to grandiosity, I must reflect on what brought me to this point. What has been given joyfully, with love, must be passed on without reservation and without expectation. For as I grow, I find that no matter how much I give with love, I receive much more in spirit.[11]

Throughout the Big Book and other A.A. literature are spiritual concepts, principles, axioms that are designed to be considered as the alcoholic moves through the spiritual transformation that is anticipated by the Twelve Steps. These address challenges that occur frequently for alcoholics, who typically arrive with significant and troubling histories. Resentment, dishonesty, self-centeredness, and fear are addressed several times, with the intention of changing the response patterns to engender instead their opposites, returning the alcoholic to acceptance, faith, and humility. In my experience, alcoholics are not unique. The nonaddicted person also carries the burdens of resentment, self-centeredness, dishonesty, fear, the need to

---

11. *Daily Reflections*, 276 and 279.

control, and the desire to appear superior. The difference is that for the addicted person, sobriety (and therefore life) depends on working on a spirituality that results in emotional health and serenity. The nonaddicted person can go a lifetime and never do the work of self-reflection necessary to identify self-destructive patterns of behavior, deal with resentment and fear, or accept responsibility for their part in conflict. My goal for the following chapters is to examine some of these spiritual principles as they might be applied to anyone who desires to grow spiritually.

Such spirituality represents major changes in a person's life: from self-focus to service, from isolation to community, from denial and lying to rigorous honesty, from fear to acceptance, from manipulation of others to making amends for inappropriate behavior, from dependence on ego-inflating crutches to recovery! This is not an easy spirituality. It requires hard work—"go to meetings, get a sponsor, work the Steps." It is a spirituality that requires commitment and surrender. Thus we find in that portion of the Big Book often read at the beginning of meetings the following:

> If you have decided you want what we have and are willing to go to any length to get it—then you are ready to take certain steps. At some of these we balked. We thought we could find an easier, softer way. But we could not. With all the earnestness at our command, we beg of you to be fearless and thorough from the start. Some of us have tried to hold on to our old ideas and the result was nil until we let go absolutely. (58)

CHAPTER 4

God of Our Understanding

Cape Cod Is Not the Ocean

FROM 1985 TO 1998 I served as the Rector (senior pastor) of Trinity Church in downtown Buffalo. Tom Heath, who had served as Rector some fifteen years previous, had a metaphor he used to describe his understanding about God—a metaphor that several parishioners shared with me which reflects how powerful this metaphor is.

Tom had a summer cabin on Cape Cod. He shared about his cabin, "I know the cape where my cabin is located. I know the tidal pools where I can find specimens at low tide. I know how the weather can roll in, when a Nor'easter is approaching. I know the best time of day to fish and the changes the seasons bring. I know where I can swim and where the bottom is too rough or the waves too dangerous. But I cannot say that I know the Atlantic Ocean or all the oceans in the world. My knowledge ends a few hundred yards from my cabin."

And he continued, "Such is my knowledge of God. I know something of God from my experience, but to say I have full or complete knowledge about God is as foolish as saying I know the oceans of the world because of my experience on Cape Cod."

This metaphor reflects the beginning premise in all theology. God is beyond our knowing, even beyond the ability of language to describe. Thus all knowledge of God is at best partial and all language about God is meta-phorical. Critics of biblical religion often critique this faith for its belief in a God who is essentially like a human father who cares for his children. The

43

fact that believers use metaphors like "Father" to describe their experience of a God who is compassionate and desires what is best for them does not mean they literally believe this analogy. I do not personally know anyone who believes God is masculine, lives in heaven—which is a place above the sky—or created the world and the cosmos in 144 hours. Believers use metaphorical language because that is the only language available to describe that which is beyond knowing. Consider the words the religious use to describe God: omnipotent, omniscient, omnipresent, eternal, Creator, and infinite. The words alone clarify that God is beyond knowing. Considering the vastness of the material world, those who believe in God understand that God must be boundless, but the words used to describe God inevitably fail to express a limitless reality.

I lived in Buffalo for thirteen years. Whenever people came to visit, we went to Niagara Falls. Every time I went to the falls, I was amazed, even overwhelmed, by their magnitude. My mind was unable to comprehend the amount of water, the strength of the current, the noise, the mist, and the size. So each time I returned, Niagara Falls was newly spectacular. All aspects of the water flow and the falls are measurable, but because they vastly exceeded my normal experience, my mind was unable to comprehend in such a way that the next visit was not filled with surprise and wonder. So when I try to imagine a "Being" without limits, I know such a concept is beyond our capacity to understand. And yet I, and many others, experience something that is beyond our understanding and that has power to transform our lives—this power we call God. Our experience is at best like a small tidal pool relative to the ocean, but the transformation of lives is clear and dramatic.

My professor of apologetic theology used to say that the only true beliefs one holds are those we are compelled to believe by evidence. Of course that evidence is not only objective, scientific, verifiable evidence; it is also the evidence of our personal experience. In areas of faith, the heart is far more important than the intellect. Faith is about experience and relationships, not unfeeling intellect and objectivity.

Spiritual Experience

It seems to me that if we seek an understanding of faith that is pragmatic rather than theoretical, then the place to start is with the recognition that the nature of God is beyond our understanding. What we truly know is our experience. While the existence of God is not verifiable, the experience of the Sacred can be very powerful and transforming. I suggest that the validity of an experience of the Transcendent lies with the reality of the person's change.

We need look no further for an example than the experience Bill W. had in Townes Hospital. Following the stock market crash of 1929, Bill's drinking went out of control. Despite arrests, missed opportunities and obligations, clear warnings from Dr. Silkworth, and despite personal resolve, Bill continued to slip. Following an intervention from his old drinking buddy Ebby (now sober as a result of a religious experience) and a visit to the Mission of Calvary Church, Bill discovered he had a desire to live. He checked himself into Townes Hospital to dry out. Three days later, after another visit from Ebby, Bill found his depression deepening. Despite having resolved that he would never be religious and without belief in a God, he suddenly found himself crying out, "If there is a God, let Him show Himself! I am ready to do anything, anything!" Then, as he tells it, this is what happened:

> Suddenly the room lit up with a great white light. I was caught up into an ecstasy which there are no words to describe. It seemed to me, in the mind's eye, that I was on a mountain and that a wind not of air but of spirit was blowing. And then it burst upon me that I was a free man. Slowly the ecstasy subsided. I lay on the bed, but now for a time I was in another world, a new world of consciousness. All about me and through me there was a wonderful feeling of Presence, and I thought to myself, "So this is the God of the preachers!" A great peace stole over me.[1]

In his earliest telling of his story, Bill quickly sped past this experience. He had learned that recounting it hindered his credibility and did not help others connect with the program. Some modern critics question if the experience might have been induced by drugs he was taking. While it is easy to be skeptical, clearly something happened. We know because we know the results. Dr. Silkworth declared without qualifications that "Unless [the alcoholic] can experience an entire psychic change there is very little hope of his recovery" (xxix). While Bill's experience is clearly subjective, the reality of what happened is seen in his total psychic change. He himself even questioned if this was real. Could it have been a hallucination as a result of his obsession with Ebby's sobriety? He called the doctor, shared

1. Bill W., *Alcoholics Anonymous Comes of Age*, 63.

in detail what had happened, and asked if it was real. After several probing questions, Dr. Silkworth responded that Bill was perfectly sane. Then he concluded, "I am but a simple man of science. Whatever it is you've got now, hang on to it because it is so much better than what you had a couple of hours ago" (14).

The next day, Ebby brought Bill a copy of William James's *The Varieties of Religious Experience*. What he got from James, influenced by his own distrust of religion, is best described in his own words:

> Spiritual experiences, James thought, would have objective reality; almost like gifts from the blue, they could transform people. Some were sudden brilliant illuminations; others came on very gradually. Some flowed out of religious channels; others did not. But nearly all had the great common denominators of pain, suffering, calamity. Complete hopelessness and deflation at depth were almost always required to make the recipient ready. The significance of all this burst upon me. *Deflation at depth* – yes, that was it. Exactly that had happened to me.[2]

Bill never had another drink of alcohol. The compulsion was no longer in control. He was changed. Bill began to carry this message to other hopeless alcoholics, unsuccessfully. He was advised to preach less, share the doctor's diagnosis and prognosis, and, like Ebby, share his own experience. Six months later in Akron, Ohio, he met Dr. Bob and A.A. was begun.

"Experience" is a more complex concept than it may appear at first. Not only is the word complex—it is both a noun and a verb—but different people may experience the same events differently:

> A husband and wife were camping when the wife woke up and turned to her husband, "What do you see?"
> "I see the stars beyond number, the vast cosmos that reminds us how small we are, how insignificant we are, how we depend on the grace of a loving God or we are nothing. What do you see?"
> His wife replied, "I see that while we were asleep, someone stole our tent."

Experience is something we go through; it is an event of some kind. However, for an event to be an experience involves thought and reflection on one's feelings about, and as a result of, the event. William James defined an experience as "what I agree to attend to."[3] Aldous Huxley in a similar

2. Bill W., *Alcoholics Anonymous Comes of Age*, 64 (italics original).

3. Kurtz and Ketcham, *Experiencing Spirituality*, 29.

statement described experience as "not what happens to a [person]; but what a [person] does with what happens to him [or her]."[4]

While I was President of General Seminary in New York City, in a seminar for entering students, I would send them to visit with leaders and community organizers in some of the poorest neighborhoods in the city. Their responses were dramatically different. For one person, the experience of seeing the changes brought by the churches through community organizing opened her mind to see new ways of addressing poverty. Another recognized that among the leaders he met he could see amazingly strong spirituality despite the abject poverty. Still another said to me, "I was so afraid in the subway in the South Bronx; I was glad others were with me; I don't think I could have done this alone." Another who attended a powerful Maafa celebration at St. Paul Community Baptist Church in East New York said the experience changed his whole understanding of slavery, but he did not think he would like to experience it again. Each student had a different experience, largely as a result of his or her previous experiences, feelings, fears, and personal sense of security.

Experience is, by definition, subjective. Experience involves the spirit of a person. It may involve the senses (touch, smell, taste, sight, hearing, kinesthesia) and will include reflection about what happened—a conscious apprehension and appreciation of how the person has been influenced and changed. Sometimes it may be years before one realizes the significance of an experience. In 1960, as a high school senior, I attended a conference sponsored by the National Council of Churches on racial integration in Tennessee. I had grown up in the segregated South. I had had no contact with African Americans. The conference was about 70 percent Black and 30 percent White. This was my first experience as a minority. I was appalled and then outraged by what I learned, but immediately it made little difference in my life. Later, I realized this was an eye-opening experience and the beginning of a lifelong involvement in efforts to end racial injustice.

Experience gives us insight, but it does not mean we now know with certainty. It frees us to be open to new experiences. Having our eyes and our minds opened to new understandings leaves us open to more new understandings. We are constantly learning new things from our experiences. To truly experience an event requires openness—a willingness to change and grow. It involves being open to learning new concepts. If one lacks the courage to be open, the opportunity for experience will be lost.

4. Huxley, quoted in Kurtz and Ketcham, *Experiencing Spirituality*, 37.

The most difficult experiences there are to share are those that affect what is happening inside a person, in the deepest part of our thinking, desiring, and feeling. Our words seem incapable of making it comprehensible to another. Some experiences will always be mystifying—to ourselves and to others. When that internal experience includes a power that is beyond our understanding, a power that transforms our lives, the inadequate word we have to describe this power is "God."

I had a difficult adolescence. Today I understand that I had substituted achievement for love. I was the practically perfect teenager. I made good grades, I was an all-county basketball player, I had a paper route and saved enough money to pay my first year in college. And I was miserable. I felt worthless. No one knew me; I felt no one loved me. I imagined that I was on a very tall, very small pedestal, and everyone was looking up at me and applauding. No one was with me, and I could not come down. I thought a lot about suicide. My identity and sense of security were centered in achievement; I could not let go of success and just be human. I was in a prison, and it was going to kill me.

Two things saved my life. The first was summer church camp where no one knew my compulsion to achieve. People accepted me, and I allowed them to care for me. I did not have to be perfect; I only had to participate. It is significant that I have no friends today from my high school years, but I met my wife at church camp, and we still have friends we visit with regularly from those camp experiences.

The second event that saved my life was an experience of God, an experience that was so personal I did not talk about it publically until I was in my mid-fifties. It happened one evening as I lay in bed contemplating suicide. A light entered the room and reached out to me. I find I am unable to explain what happened beyond that, but I knew I was loved. At the heart of the universe there was love, love that knew my name, that cared for me, that wanted for me what was best for me. Several years later, I discovered the work of the theologian Paul Tillich, and his words described what I had experienced: though I felt worthless and unacceptable, I was accepted and loved by God and others, and all I needed to do was accept that I was acceptable. One might ask: Was this truly an external event or was it internal? Was this experience created by me because of my needs? Was I dreaming? I do not believe there is an objective answer to these questions. What I do know is my life changed. In spite of many challenges and failures, I have never lacked confidence that I have worth. As a friend of mine says,

"God loves you; how dare you not love yourself." Or as I learned in the Twelve-Step community, "God don't make junk." Whatever happened, it was a spiritual experience that brought healing, freedom, and change; and it has lasted a lifetime. This experience was and is beyond my understanding, it was something that transformed my life. I am comfortable calling this power that changed me "God."

God is beyond our knowing, even beyond the ability of language to describe. All knowledge of God is at best partial, and all language about God is metaphorical. Any concept we have of God is like saying we know about the ocean because we know a cove off Cape Cod. Our concepts are too small. Those of us who accept this premise talk about God humbly, use "I statements," and speak primarily from our personal experience. Though I understand that the Steps refer to "God as we understand him" in order clearly to avoid theological controversy, mentally I like to translate this to *God of our experience*. And experiences vary greatly among many different people.

All of this does not mean that whatever a person identifies as a "spiritual experience" is authentic. At times when I am speaking to A.A. gatherings, I ask the question: How many were "saved" and drank again? A lot of hands go up. I believe many alcoholics at some point in their progression into alcoholism bargain with God, seeking a God who will solve their problems, rather than accepting their own powerlessness and, with that acceptance, discovering a God who is known in our powerlessness. We must always be humble, even tentative, when discussing spiritual experience since it involves not only the events but also the perception, the mindfulness, the feelings, and the assumptions of the person. Despite this subjective quality, I believe there are some characteristics that differentiate some experiences, pointing toward the legitimacy of a particular experience.

The first characteristic is the effect such an experience has had on a person. Bill W.'s experience had an immediate and dramatic effect. He was freed from the compulsion to drink. One symptom of the disease of alcoholism or other addictions is the loss of the ability to choose. The compulsion to drink and the inability to drink in moderation leave the person powerless. The spiritual experience gave Bill, as it has given millions of others, the power to choose.

If we accept the premise that "a religious, or spiritual experience is the act of giving up reliance on one's own omnipotence,"[5] then a second

5. Dr. Harry Tiebout, quoted in Bill W., *Language of the Heart*, 99.

characteristic of such an experience is gaining the ability to ask for help. The experience that we are unable to help ourselves gives way to a new perspective. Though we cannot help ourselves, we can be helped if we will accept the help of a power beyond ourselves. Bill discovered this new reality in his conversation with Dr. Bob. Not only did Dr. Bob need help; Bill also needed Dr. Bob's assistance. A.A. was founded on this spiritual premise: Together we can do what we were unable to do alone; acceptance of one's limitations opens a door to accept help from others.

A third characteristic can be found in the long-lasting effect of the change. The example of Ebby T. reminds us that what was clearly a transforming spiritual experience may not last forever. There is a need to nurture the new life continually. One can only wonder what would have happened to Bill W. if he had not found Dr. Bob and discovered the mutual relationship of a shared struggle. Some see the chain of events in Akron as a continuation of the divine intervention of Bill's spiritual experience. Bill's despair lead to the phone call from the Mayflower Hotel to Calvary Church, which led to ten calls to members of the Oxford Group before he reached Norman Shepherd, who put him in touch with Henrietta Seiberling, who invited him to her home and set up the appointment with Dr. Bob. The genius of Alcoholics Anonymous is to have tied together spiritual experience and the recovering community.

These three aspects of a spiritual experience have been true for me as well. The support from the church community has meant that my single spiritual experience has provided a lifetime of freedom. And my involvement with Alcoholics Anonymous has provided a community with further spiritual growth in which the nonreligious language has provided new insights into my personal experience and for my ministry.

In A.A., the spiritual experience is one of healing. On the one hand, we experience that we are unable to help ourselves; and on the other hand, we experience that we can be helped if we will accept the help of a power beyond ourselves. On the one hand, we discover our basic identity as limited human beings; on the other hand, we are invited into new relationships in a healing community. We do not have to get involved in theology or philosophy about the existence or the nature of God. One's Higher Power is what works. Period. It does not matter if one's understanding of God is a traditional theistic view, or if it is the biblical view of a king on the throne above the sky, or if it is simply Mystery, or if (as with Native Americans) it is of a Creator, or if it is simply the power of the group—if it works to keep one from taking a drink today, it is that person's Higher Power. This pragmatic understanding is the point where we begin to develop an understanding of secular spirituality.

As noted in the previous chapter, the Big Book makes clear that what we are calling "spiritual experience" is not always dramatic. The more common experience develops slowly over a period of time. Often the experience comes as a result of the changes that have happened to the individual. A profound alteration in the person's life has taken place in a remarkably short time. How has this happened? Such change hardly seems to be the result of personal, individual effort, since such efforts have a history of failure. Many members find that they have tapped an unsuspected inner resource which they identify with their own conception of a Power greater than themselves.

Alcoholics Anonymous is a spiritual program, not because it affirms the existence of God or any theology about God. It is not a religion. It is a spiritual program because at its center is the affirmation of mystery at how one alcoholic sharing with another brings hope and transformation. There are many kinds of spiritual experience. All of them, whatever form they take, have one effect: They make a person capable of doing something they could not do before. Bill W., reflecting much later on his own experience and his conversation with Dr. Bob, sums them up simply, "Thus I was set free. It was just as simple, yet just as mysterious, as that."[6]

Hearts Touched

When an alcoholic walks through the door the first time to attend an A.A. meeting, when the same alcoholic hears her story on the lips of the speaker at the meeting and hears the laughter and sees someone who is healthy, joyous, and free; when this alcoholic connects her life with that of the speaker and also sees the difference, then that spark of hope is born—perhaps it is possible to have a sober life. That hope is the beginning of a faith that life can be better. That faith will develop through relationships. When a person comes back to a second meeting that is an act of faith. The person returns with hope and the growing recognition that this is a place she belongs. It is not an intellectual conclusion; it is a heart that has been touched.

Faith is relational; faith is born when the heart is touched; faith is not anti-intellectual; it is nonintellectual. Because faith is relational and is born

6. Bill W., *Language of the Heart*, 198.

when the emotions are affected, it is often caught from another person. Most active alcoholics come to A.A. out of the despair of a life that has become unmanageable. The stories I have heard about individuals' first A.A. meetings rarely recount what was said; most do not remember. Nor do these first meetings seem to be moments of immediate spiritual enlightenment. Many remember being surprised by the amount of laughter, but mostly their stories describe themselves as a person in need, recognizing that recovery is possible with help, getting phone numbers from other members, and resolving to come back. Somehow, in the identification with the speaker or with other members, hope is born. That spark of hope and the welcoming from the members of the group mark the beginning of a change. Important words are spoken, "Keep coming back. Get a sponsor. Work the Steps." When the still-suffering alcoholic keeps coming back and gets a sponsor, then the process of spiritual growth begins by working the Steps, and a life is changed.

I served for over thirty years as a parish pastor. For the first few years I was a compassionate enabler. I would receive a call at 2:00 in the morning from someone who had had a few glasses of wine and "needed" to talk. I would get up and go to their home. I would listen with all my listening skills. I would help them rationalize and feel better. I helped take away the pain that might have led to change. I felt good about myself, but there were two problems: first, nothing changed in their lives, and second, sometimes they did not even remember I had been there.

Later, when I began to be informed about this cunning, baffling, and powerful disease, I decided that I was the new savior of drunks. I knew the symptoms, I knew the solution (A.A.), and I would get those in trouble into the program. One time an oncoming car ran off the road into the ditch and flipped on its side. I helped the driver, who reeked of alcohol, get out of the car, took him home, and talked with his wife about alcoholism. I returned later to share with both of them information I had about A.A. They were pleasant, but when I offered to take him to an A.A. meeting or her to Al-Anon, they were certain that would not be necessary. I left some literature for them to read. To the best of my knowledge, my visit had absolutely no effect.

A short time later, I was pulling out of a parking lot, when a car turned into the lot and headed straight toward me. My horn blowing made no difference. He plowed directly into my car—totaled it! He was so drunk he could not get out of the driver's seat for some time. By the time the police arrived, however, he and his wife had managed to change seats. The policeman indicated he had not seen him driving, so he would not give him a ticket for DWI. I had a feeling this had happened before. I got their address from the police report and took A.A. literature to their home. Again, to the best of my knowledge, my visit had absolutely no effect.

There were other attempts, until finally I learned I am unable to be the savior. I only had information about the disease. Information does not give a person who is suffering that spark of hope that will lead them to the A.A. Fellowship. Information is aimed at the head; hope comes when the heart is touched. And hearts are touched when the suffering alcoholic hears their story on the lips of someone who has been there and has found a new life. So I learned a new way to respond to the still-suffering alcoholic, a way that has actually helped over the years. As a pastor, I would receive a call when someone was in crisis. I would then call a friend in A.A., and together we would visit the family. I would talk with the nondrinking spouse about the disease, and the friend would share their story with the suffering alcoholic. I learned, as A.A. #3 (Bill D.) said, "people who talked to me wanted to help me, and my pride prevented me from listening to them" (185). What is needed is the sharing by someone who has lived in the chaos of addiction and with whom the alcoholic can identify. Only when hearts are touched can hope be born.

I have a good friend who says she remembers only one thing from her first meeting. She was told, "You will never have to face your problem alone again." Her heart was touched. That kept her coming back; we just celebrated her thirty-second year of sobriety.

An old-timer said it this way:

> At my very first AA meeting . . . I heard words of love, understanding and compassion . . . I believe the hand of God reached down at that meeting and healed me. For from that day thirty-eight years ago to this, I have not had a desire to drink or escape from reality again.[7]

A young person, new to A.A., described it this way:

> I opened the door and walked into the warmth, the laughter, the acceptance, and the love that is AA. No one asked me who I was or what I wanted; no one asked me how much money I had or what I did for a living; no one asked me where I did my drinking or what my sexual preferences were. The smiling man who greeted me told

7. Pauline B., "From Handcuffs to Hope," 19.

me that night that if I thought I had a drinking problem, I was in the right place.[8]

This may sound like all one must do is show up at a meeting and allow the spirit to restore their sanity, but we know it is not that simple. Yes, one may be touched at a first meeting; one may feel connected; and hope may be born, however weak. But they must come back again and again, and they must take some risks with the group. To turn one's will and life over to the God of our understanding involves the risk of being vulnerable and honest with the group. Such risk is a kind of leap of faith, and without it one will never know the power of the Fellowship. The Spirit of God is embodied in the group.

My friend Bill had attended several meetings, but he still did not say much; he still sat in the back of the room. He was not drinking, but he did not feel connected to the group. He wondered if he would keep coming back. He got a ride home from the meeting. In the car, the driver asked, "What are you planning to do tonight?" Bill responded, "I don't know; I need to relax a bit; I think I may smoke a little pot." The friend responded, "In A.A. we don't use other drugs." Bill says he only heard one word in that sentence—"we." "We in A.A." From that moment Bill says he identified; he was a member of A.A., and thus his spiritual journey began.

To know the power of the God of our understanding, one must take that step of being vulnerable in the group, of sharing personal history, accepting weakness, and humbly asking God to remove shortcomings. Father Dowling described A.A. as "a democracy of people helping through mutual vulnerability."[9] Faith involves a kind of risk, a leap of faith. Faith is relational and cannot be experienced outside of trust. Bill said it in chapter 5: "Rarely have we seen a person fail who has thoroughly followed our path. Those who do not recover are people who cannot or will not completely give themselves to this simple program" (58).

Faith, trust, is not anti-intellectual; it is nonintellectual. Allow me to illustrate. If I say to you that my wife loves me, there is no way I can prove that statement with objective, scientific, verifiable evidence. Her actions could have many different motives, and what one person sees as disinterested could also be seen as giving needed freedom. Similar actions can be interpreted differently. I cannot prove she loves me. There might be evidence that she does not love me, such as infidelity, repeated lying, or

8. J. B., "Above All, an Alcoholic," 28.

9. Fitzgerald, *Soul of Sponsorship*, 105.

constant unexplained absence; but there is never irrefutable evidence she loves me. The only way I can know she loves me is to trust that she loves me. In trust, I can see how her actions are loving, caring, and demonstrate concern for our relationship and for my best interest. If trust is broken, then I will give different motives to her actions. We cannot know love or help or appropriate critique from an objective point of view; we can only know the other and their concern for us when we take that leap of faith and trust the love is present.

Similarly, for the recovering alcoholic to know the power found in the Twelve-Step program, they, having found hope, must grow more trusting of others and more accepting of working the Steps. No one can earn another's trust. To trust involves a kind of leap of faith. It is born when the heart is touched. The only God in which we can have faith is the God who has touched our hearts. All the debate about what we ought to believe is irrelevant. The God that we have experienced is the only God that matters, the God that changes our lives. And this God is at work in so many different aspects of our lives.

Our experience of God may be—probably is—as small as the knowledge of a small stream is in comparison with all the rivers, lakes, and oceans in the world, but it can lead to a faith that transforms our lives. When that faith leads us into a community of truth, healing, and spiritual and emotional growth, that results in a transformation. There are not a lot of answers; no certainty; only a lot of ambiguity. We humans desire more certainty. When I look at my own spiritual journey over the years, I see many, many changes in my understanding of God, of how God relates to this world, and of what is the divine will for me. When I share my insights with others, that diversity increases. Ironically, part of what we must surrender when we embrace faith is this desire for certainty. We must learn to live with ambiguity.

But as we live in relationship with the faith community, we grow in love, in freedom, and in insight. The spirituality of the Twelve Steps depends not on an understanding about God, but on the indispensable spiritual qualities of "willingness, honesty, and open mindedness" (568). Such is the pragmatic faith found in the Fellowship of Alcoholics Anonymous; such is our knowledge of a Power greater than ourselves that brings serenity. We live with ambiguity about God—perhaps I should say mystery, but in those in recovery we have visible, verifiable results of a power beyond our understanding. That is enough.

CHAPTER 5

Truth as Dialogue

Doubt is not a pleasant condition, but certainty is an absurd one.

—Voltaire[1]

WOULD ANYONE BELIEVE AN Asian American Harvard graduate could be an outstanding NBA player? It seems an unlikely combination, but assumptions can be misleading.

Jeremy Shu-How Lin grew up in the San Francisco Bay area and was voted Northern California Player of the Year his senior year in high school, but did not receive any athletic scholarship offers from universities. So he went to Harvard where he was three times selected as the all-conference player for the Ivy League. He was not selected in the NBA draft, but was able to secure a contract with his hometown Golden State Warriors in 2010. Following a year with little playing time, he was let go by the Warriors and was picked up by the New York Knicks as their number four point guard. In February 2012, the Knicks were having a disastrous season, having lost eleven of their last thirteen games. Lin had only played fifty-five minutes in their first twenty-three games. On February 4, however, Lin's coach finally put him in the game, primarily because every other point guard was injured. He led the Knicks to an upset victory over the New Jersey Nets. He led the Knicks to victory in the next seven games in which he started. In early February the Knicks had considered releasing him, and he had decided that if he was released, he would quit basketball altogether.

1. https://www.quotes.net/quote/6752.

Daryl Morey, the general manager of the Houston Rockets, who was experimenting with computer analysis for selecting players, who rated Lin via this analytical approach as a top pick but who passed him by in the draft in 2010 and again in 2011, refers to the failure to draft Lin as "confirmation bias."[2] Confirmation bias depends on the natural tendency for the human mind to see what it expects to see and to miss seeing what it does not expect. Thus when one has an opinion, then the evidence is arranged to support that opinion. Evidence supporting the opinion is upheld while evidence that does not support it is diminished. In other words, if one thinks an Asian American Harvard graduate does not sound like a basketball player, then evidence will be arranged to support this premature conclusion. Confirmation bias is insidious because it happens without the person realizing it is happening.

The mind is not a passive receiver of reality. There is, for example, a major challenge to teach robots to see, to recognize different things—like the difference between a cake, a pie, a wheel, a tire, a frisbee, a dish. They're all round circles, but are dramatically different. We have no trouble making such distinctions, because our brain does something marvelous—it sorts and assigns meaning, automatically.

We don't see things as if they were just a bunch of dots on a screen. Without thinking, we know the difference between a tire and a cake, because the mind automatically shapes and sorts the data the eye (or the ear) receives based on our experience, our personal interests, and our presuppositions. Without such sorting we would be unable to function. Such sorting, however, goes beyond recognition of what an object is. We sort what is threatening, what is affirming, what will make us sad, what will make us feel welcome, what seems truthful. Just as we automatically recognize a wheel, so too we automatically recognize a basketball player or a computer geek on the basis of our experience and our emotional/spiritual history and the community in which we reside. We do not see reality as it is; rather the mind actively shapes the data it receives. Thus we say people perceive the world through lenses. Even when seeking to be objective and honest, pure truth is elusive.

Confirmation bias is not the only way we filter the data we perceive without conscious intent. For example, we are more conscious of negative factors in our lives than positive, as a result of both experience and biological predisposition. This explains the common advice given to those who

2. Lewis, *Undoing Project*, 40.

would invest in the stock market—when the market drops is not the time to sell. People who sell find that they generally lose more money than if they had done nothing. This advice is needed because fear of loss is greater than the expectation that waiting can bring gain. We are wired to find and react to threats and setbacks. Imagine animals looking for food—they live a life of eat-or-be-eaten. They are much more likely to respond to the threat of a predator than to the opportunity to seize a meal. The reason is obvious. If they miss the meal, there will be other opportunities; if they fail to react to a predator, there may be no future. The primitive mind (dominated by the thalamus and the amygdala) is part of the human mind, and it provides the first responses. Thus we are more likely to react to bad events more quickly, strongly, and persistently than to equivalent good events. As a result, avoidance of negative experiences overpowers objective evaluation.[3] Thus we recognize why fear is such a strong force in our lives.

Then there is that universal practice of seeing others' weaknesses and faults but not your own. When we make comparisons with others, we set them up to favor ourselves. Thus a study of such "unconscious overclaiming" showed that when husbands and wives estimated the percentage of housework each does, their estimates totaled over 120 percent. In a similar study with MBA students, when they estimated their contribution to the team, the estimates totaled over 139 percent.[4]

Jonathan Haidt uses the image of riding a elephant to illustrate this phenomenon. The elephant represents the primitive mind, which is in control, operating automatically under its fight-flight logic, and the thinking part of the brain, the frontal cortex, rides along thinking it is in control, which occasionally it is. All our perception is shaped by these unconscious biases.

Kahneman and Tversky

Daniel Kahneman and Amos Tversky were two Israeli psychologists who began collaborating together while they served on the faculty of Hebrew University. Between 1971 and 1979 they published a series of papers that developed scientific insight into why and how the mind misjudges. These papers established the field of behavioral economics, the combination of economics and psychology. For this and subsequent work Daniel

3. Haidt, *Happiness Hypothesis*, 28–29.
4. Haidt, *Happiness Hypothesis*, 69.

Kahneman was awarded the Nobel Prize in economics in 2002, six years after his collaborator had died.[5]

Their focus was on human error. Why do rational people make poor decisions? Are there patterns to such poor decisions that can be discerned? If so, can we learn from them in order to make better decisions?

Kahneman and Tversky started their research investigating apparent anomalies and contradictions in human behavior. For example, as Kahneman says, people may drive across town to save $5 on a $15 calculator but not drive across town to save $5 on a $125 coat. In another example subjects when offered a choice formulated in one way might display risk aversion but when offered essentially the same choice formulated in a different way might display risk-seeking behavior. In the early 1980s, to treat cancer there were two options: surgery or radiation. Surgery was more likely to extend one's life, but it also had a small risk of death on the operating table. When patients were told they had a 90 percent chance of surviving surgery, 82 percent opted for surgery. But when they were told they had a 10 percent chance of dying from surgery, only 54 percent chose surgery! Again, the framing of the data influenced its valuation.

Kahneman gives another example where some Americans were offered insurance against their own death in a terrorist attack while on a trip to Europe, while another group were offered insurance that would cover death of any kind on the trip. The former group were willing to pay more even though "death of any kind" includes "death in a terrorist attack." Kahneman suggests that the attribute of fear is being substituted for a calculation of the total risks of travel. Fear of terrorism for these subjects was stronger than a general fear of dying on a foreign trip.

They developed a series of "heuristics" to describe nonlogical ways we human beings make decisions. A heuristic is a judgment shortcut that generally get us where we need to go quickly, but at the cost of occasionally sending us off course. Heuristics are useful because they simplify decision-making and reduce the required effort.

A couple of examples will suffice.

"Representativeness" describes how we make decisions regarding the likelihood of a specific outcome for events that are uncertain, like success in a new job, the outcome of an election, or the state of the stock market. The mind does not do the hard work of articulating all the factors involved and

---

5. A recent popular account of the work of Kahneman and Tversky is found in Lewis, *Undoing Project*.

calculating the odds of each and then assessing relative importance of each factor in order to make a final decision. Rather, Kahneman and Tversky argued that we make such judgments by comparing the current event with a model we have developed in our minds. In their earliest paper they did not address how these models are developed, but in later publications it is clear they represent our past experience, what we have been taught, and how we imagine such a scenario. The more a storm cloud appears to look like clouds that have brought rain in the past, the more likely we are to take actions in preparation for rain. The more a basketball player looks like our mental model of an NBA player, the more likely we will think him to be an NBA player. Often the decisions based on what is "representative" of the model in one's mind are correct, but at times mistakes are made. Kahneman and Tversky recognized these were not random mistakes. Through testing they determined that these mistakes were systematic, they were the result of shortcuts to decision-making.

Not all decisions are as inconsequential as rain storms or the NBA draft. In October 1973, Egypt attacked Israel in what became known as the Yom Kippur War. After the war, intensive analysis of why Israel was caught off guard discerned that Israeli intelligence had insisted, despite a lot of evidence to the contrary, that Egypt would never attack Israel so long as Israel maintained air superiority. This assumption regarding air superiority represented a model of future events in the minds of those in intelligence such that they simply did not see the danger in Egypt's mobilizing.

There are also factors that impact our estimations that are based on information that is not relevant. Take for example, the phenomena of "Anchoring." The best way to understand it is to use two of the tests Kahneman and Tversky used. They gave a group of high school students the following math problem and only five seconds in which to solve it:

$$8 \times 7 \times 6 \times 5 \times 4 \times 3 \times 2 \times 1 = ?$$

Obviously the students would have to guess as five seconds is not long enough to actually do the math. Then they gave a second set of students a similar problem also with only five seconds to form their guess:

$$1 \times 2 \times 3 \times 4 \times 5 \times 6 \times 7 \times 8 = ?$$

One would expect the two group's answers to be close, but they were dramatically and statistically different. The first group's median answer was 2,250; the second group's median answer was 512; the correct answer is

40,320. The reason Kahneman and Tversky gave for the difference is that the first group was tied (anchored) to the number 8 while the second group started with and was tied to the number 1.

Perhaps an even better example of anchoring is found in an experiment where volunteers spun a wheel (like the wheel of fortune) with numbers ranging from one to one hundred. They were then asked to estimate the percentage of African countries in the United Nations. People who spun a higher number on the wheel tended to guess a higher percentage, and those who spun a lower number guessed a lower percentage! The participants' answers were influenced by the number they spun on the wheel—a totally unrelated number. The number on the wheel anchored their mind to think in terms of higher or lower numbers.

Human beings make decisions. We do not like uncertainty, and the mind is the tool we have to make sense out of a world that is filled with uncertainty. We evolved long before the tools of statistics, logic, and computers became available. So human beings developed shortcuts, rules of thumb, to allow us to make decisions. We think we are being rational; Kahneman and Tversky make clear we are using shortcuts that are often right, but are also at times wrong. We think of our mistakes as random; Kahneman and Tversky show us that they are systematic. In other words, errors are not only common, they are also predictable. In short, our brain is programmed so that we cannot know fully the circumstances in which we operate, and therefore we make mistakes. We cannot know the truth.

This is different from the parable of the blind men and the elephant.[6] In that parable, each man, touching a different part of the elephant, had a different experience of what an elephant is like; however, each man had a true experience. The problem illustrated by the parable is that we have partial experiences of reality, but by sharing the different experiences we can arrive at the truth. Kahneman's and Tversky's thesis is not that we have a partial, but true, understanding of reality; their thesis is that as individuals we cannot know truth in complex situations because our minds

---

6. Six blind men, who do not know what an elephant looks like, each feel a different part of the elephant's body, but only one part. They then describe the elephant based on their limited experience and their descriptions of the elephant are different from each other. The first person, whose hand lands on the trunk, says, "This being is like a thick snake." To another whose hand reaches the ear, it seems like a kind of fan. The man whose hand is upon its leg says, "the elephant is a pillar like a tree trunk." The one who places his hand upon its side says the elephant "is a wall." Another who feels its tail describes it as a rope. The last feels its tusk, and states that the elephant is hard and smooth, like a spear.

are programmed to use heuristics (shortcuts) in order to make decisions quickly.

In the pursuit of truth, seeking to force people to share their feelings, hopes, disappointments, and struggles is inappropriate and abusive. Such truth can only be received humbly and reverently.

> A man was riding his motorcycle along a California beach when suddenly the sky clouded above his head and, in a booming voice, the Lord said, "Because you have TRIED to be faithful to me in all ways, I will grant you one wish."
>
> The biker pulled over and said, "Build a bridge to Hawaii so I can ride over anytime I want."
>
> The Lord said, "Your request is materialistic: think of the enormous challenges for that kind of undertaking: the supports required to reach the bottom of the Pacific and the concrete and steel it would take! It will nearly exhaust several natural resources. I can do it, but it is hard for me to justify your desire for worldly things. Take a little more time and think of something that could possibly help mankind."
>
> The biker thought about it for a long time. Finally, he said, "Lord, I wish that I and all men could understand our wives; I want to know how she feels inside, what she's thinking when she gives me the silent treatment, why she cries, what she means when she says nothing's wrong, and how I can make a woman truly happy."
>
> The Lord replied, "You want two lanes or four on that bridge?"[7]

As difficult as it is for one to know the truth, we cannot abandon the search for truth. For the alcoholic, the need to accept the truth (that he or she is addicted and the addiction is making life unmanageable) is the difference between life and death. While the consequences of our ignoring the need for truth are usually less dramatic, our actions do have consequences, and when based on intentional ignorance or false understandings those consequences are often destructive.

Human beings are spiritual beings. As spiritual beings we are in the process of developing our spirituality throughout our lives until death or mental deterioration. Development of a healthy spirituality depends on seeking and accepting truth about oneself. Steps Four (make a fearless moral inventory), Five (share it with God and another human being), and Six and Seven (ask God to remove our character defects) all point to the difficult task of knowing oneself. While these steps appear to suggest an

---

7. Kurtz and Ketcham, *Experiencing Spirituality*, 37–38.

evaluation of one's negative history and qualities, in practice, evaluation of positive and often neglected characteristics is also included. All of us, if we want to grow, need to know the problems that need cleaning up and the assets that need further development. This is hard work. It involves an earnest seeking to know the truth about oneself. As Step Five suggests, this may well necessitate sharing with another who will be part of one's self-discovery. Failure to be open to the truth—unpleasant or affirming—will lead to arresting one's spiritual growth. We all have a concept of who we are. The only option is whether our self-concept is accurate or distorted. Seeking the truth about oneself, as difficult as that task is to do, is the virtue that leads to healthy spiritual growth.

Truth is also a primary tool for the settling of differences. Two economists have opposing views on what are the best policies for moving toward full employment while preventing runaway inflation. In an ideal world in which neither person is defensive, they could together develop a list of agreed-upon facts that are relevant to the problem and then reach some mutual conclusions. Further, as they move forward in time, they can evaluate and modify their original conclusions based on new information. This is idealized because it assumes two people who are searching for objective truth. This is the way we solve problems.

To abandon the search for factual information is to abandon personal spiritual growth and the possibility of development of rational policies for civil society. To abandon the search for factual information is to abandon freedom. If nothing is true, if there are no facts, then no one can criticize power, because there is no basis upon which to do so. If nothing is true, then all is spectacle. The biggest wallet pays for the most blinding lights. If facts cannot be recognized and agreed upon, then there is no way to debate, no way to listen and understand, no way to question and disagree, no way to develop appropriate policies, plans, and responses. Cultivating the habits of an open mind and being willing to entertain new or unpopular ideas, while also holding to one's own values and perspective, is the pathway to truth. The current polarization in our society tells us we need some new tools to assist us with this task.

A Twelve-Step Approach to Truth

Yes, alcoholics hide their excessive drinking from others; but even more they need to blind themselves to the reality of the progressing condition.

The ability to rationalize, justify, and blame in order to avoid responsibility is finely tuned. Lying becomes the norm for relationships, but even more for one's own self-awareness. The following statements are just a few I have heard over the years:

> "It did not make sense that I was powerless over something I should be able to control."

> "The more the disease affected other parts of my life, the harder I fought for control in those areas."

> "I would do anything to hurt anyone who threatened my view of myself as a responsible adult. They were wrong; I could not be an alcoholic."

> "As the disease progressed, I found it impossible to share my sense of strangeness with anyone. The inability to express something critically important about oneself is profoundly alienating, but with more alcohol that alienation seemed to dissolve. When drinking I felt more connected and no longer crazy, back in control of my life. I drank to get in control of myself, yet my drinking was out of control."

> "When I got my third DWI, I thought I was just unlucky that the policeman was on the road I was taking home."

As a whole, few groups struggle with knowing the truth as much as active alcoholics. This is part of the reason intervention in the disease is so difficult. Present-day science now has demonstrated that addiction is a brain disease; the brain becomes programmed so the alcoholic feels they will die if they do not get their drink, or that some other bad outcome will result. Getting the alcohol/drug becomes the most important thing in their life, becomes an obsession. But being focused compulsively on drinking is not acceptable—not acceptable in our culture, not acceptable to the alcoholic who wants to think of him or herself as responsible, not acceptable to family, friends, and cohorts. So the alcoholic creates a psychic edifice using blame, lies, rationalizations, filters, and diminishments. These distortions are further fueled by episodes of loss of memory (i.e., blackouts) that sometimes occur with inebriation. The power of denial for the active alcoholic makes honest acceptance of their addiction very difficult.

Not surprisingly, the focus in Twelve-Step spirituality on rigorous honesty is seen as essential to recovery. Chapter 4 in *Alcoholics Anonymous* begins with these words:

> Those who do not recover are people who cannot or will not completely give themselves to this simple program, usually men and women who are constitutionally incapable of being honest with themselves. There are such unfortunates. They are not at fault; they seem to have been born that way. They are naturally incapable of grasping and developing a manner of living which demands rigorous honesty. Their chances are less than average. There are those, too, who suffer from grave emotional and mental disorders, but many of them do recover if they have the capacity to be honest. (58)

To a lesser degree all of us are caught in denial. So add denial to the list of ways human beings are programmed to see the world through filters. Guilt, shame, ego, fear, pride, hope, prejudice, preconceptions—we do not see the world as it is. We can even add heuristics to this list. Perhaps the most difficult task we face in life is to remove our filters so as to see the world as it is and to see ourselves as we are, to see ourselves as others see us. The active alcoholic's denial magnifies this task. Given the success of Twelve-Step spirituality and the magnitude of this challenge, we can expect this program to provide us with a model for those who seek to know truth. The fact that success is achieved in the context of such powerful denial is compelling and worth examination.

(1) Letting go of denial begins with the First Step. Unless one admits there is a problem, there will be no working toward a solution. Acceptance that one has become powerless over alcohol—that life has become unmanageable—is how recovery begins. For the alcoholic this step may feel like defeat. I am powerless over my will power; I am powerless over controlling my life; I am powerless to control my self-respect. To accept as true what is obviously true to everyone else is devastating to the alcoholic's self-image. But only by accepting that life is out of control can the process of discovering one's true self begin.

For those who are not active alcoholics, we must also begin by accepting that all the things we think we know about ourselves may not be true. We must also begin by accepting that our decisions, which we think are rational, are not very rational. We also begin by recognizing that our view of reality is based on biases we have carried our entire lives. The ability to see more clearly begins with the recognition that we do not see the world as it is. Unless we recognize we have a problem, we will not begin to search for a solution. Admitting that we cannot by our own effort alone see the world and self as they truly are, admitting our powerlessness, lays the ground work for facing the self honestly. Be assured, the benefit of humbly recognizing one's limits allows for, and is even necessary for, favorable shifts in perception and experience to begin.

I enjoy reading light mysteries for escapist relaxation. The Chief Inspector Gamache Mystery series by Louise Penny offers surprising advice about how to solve a mystery, or as Inspector Gamache says, it is advice about how to discover wisdom. Regularly using these four sentences, he says, will lead to insight and wisdom:

> I don't know.
> I need help.
> I'm sorry.
> I was wrong.

When we think we know, do not want help, ignore others, and are convinced we are right, we cannot learn. Discovering truth often means having to change. Being open to truth means being open to change and being open to being changed. The search for truth begins with acceptance of our inability to know truth and seeking to know what we do not know.

(2) For the alcoholic, taking the terrifying step of accepting they are powerless over alcohol is made possible because they are now surrounded by others who have successfully taken these steps and today are living happier, healthier sober lives. Normally, meetings provide an important community context, and new members are encouraged right away to get a sponsor—someone to whom they can relate and with whom they are in frequent contact, sharing their experience with working the Steps and living sober. A sponsor ties one directly to the broad experience of the A.A. community. With the support of the sponsor and with the support of the members of the group(s), the person takes other Steps that help them to come closer to the truth. Step Four requires an active process of making a searching and fearless moral inventory—an appraisal of past actions and experiences that places the newly sober alcoholic squarely across from a version of their history, their truth, with which they likely have not previously reckoned. Subsequent Steps continue this fact-facing approach, and afford the alcoholic a method of reconciling this past through the process of admitting wrongs

(Step Five), becoming willing to change (Step Six), asking for spiritual help to change (Step Seven), and setting the past straight through making amends (Steps Eight and Nine) The individual then is set to continue the process of self-searching and responsibility on a daily basis (Step Ten). This is the path to rigorous honesty.

When a community of people who have followed this path get together, the group develops a culture that encourages honesty. Members become less fearful of negative truths; in fact, laughter is a norm as members share their own stories of disastrous events or of inflated egos. The culture of the A.A. groups I have experienced are remarkably consistent: a primary concern for the still-suffering alcoholic, an expectation that all be as honest and truthful as they are able, and love and tolerance for one another. A friend once said, "Tolerance is the art of seeing yourself as others see you—and not getting mad about it." This culture of tolerance and truthfulness is a powerful force that allows members to see themselves and their situation more clearly.

The culture in which most of us live does not strongly support tolerance and truthfulness. As a result, within our competitive, success-oriented, image-focused culture, we become defensive, prejudicial, secretive, and judgmental. These are not characteristics that help us see the truth clearly. Truth-seekers thrive in a culture that supports truth-telling, is tolerant of differences, and does not judge failure.

(3) Listening is another characteristic of A.A. meetings that supports truth-telling. If it is a speaker meeting, obviously those in attendance listen. If it is a discussion meeting, there are norms that are followed. In general, meetings do not allow cross-talk; no one interrupts or questions or debates what another member says. Each person who desires to speak is honored by the others' listening, seeking to understand and identify with the speaker. No one dominates the discussion; each person has an opportunity to share his or her insight. Listening is a kind of surrender. As a participant, I surrender my desire to be all-knowing and to be sure everyone else knows, understands, and follows my way of doing things.

> There will always be people in the Fellowship with whom I don't see eye-to-eye, but that doesn't mean we can't work together. The Fellowship wouldn't be what it is today if we always saw eye-to-eye on everything.[8]

8. Sue F., "Principles Before Personalities," 23.

I have learned to keep quiet when I disagree and to give others freedom to express opinions widely different from my own—without giving in to the urge to enlighten them. I am grateful for all the voices of AA.[9]

In the pursuit of truth, we can learn a lot by listening. Serious listening involves letting go of the self-assurance that we are right, involves hearing opposing views without seeing them as personal attacks, involves working to understand the other person, and being open to changing not only one's own ideas but also one's values and actions.

(4) Interestingly, the governance structure and process of Alcoholics Anonymous also supports careful, thorough, and respectful vetting of matters, which discerns truth and ultimately leads to better-informed decision-making. The Second Tradition ("For our group's purpose, there is but one ultimate authority—a loving God as He may express Himself in our group conscience. Our leaders are but trusted servants; they do not govern.") illustrates a core value that honors the position of the whole group over any individual person or perspective. In practice, there are a number of typical procedures that are followed that facilitate this, whether at the group, state, regional, or board level, or at the annual Conference made up of delegates from the United States and Canada, Board members, and Directors. Typically actions are only adopted with the agreement of two-thirds of the voting body. Speaking times are limited and members are asked not to speak a second time until after all who want to speak have had the opportunity. In addition, there is a profound respect for honoring and listening to the minority perspective; after a vote, those who voted with the losing side are invited to speak. Sometimes this leads to a reconsideration of the matter and even a reversal of the decision. In addition, all those who hold positions as leaders in the Fellowship are governed by a principle of rotation. Terms are strictly limited so no one gains a dominant position of leadership. Finally, there is an accepted norm that A.A. is a self-correcting organization. If any action taken this year is seen in the future as being inappropriate, it can be readdressed and changed.

As Chair of the General Service Board, and therefore as one of those who presides, I can affirm that it often took hours to reach a decision. However, in pursuit of the best decisions for the whole Fellowship, listening to

9. Eric D., "Humble Proportion," 8.

the multitude of voices was and is essential. I have come to understand that decisions made quickly often take a major effort to implement, but decisions that are thoroughly considered from a group of diverse persons take a long time to make but are implemented almost immediately.

This model offers insight for those of us who seek to know the truth but who are not part of a Twelve-Step program:

(1) We begin by accepting that we too are in denial. We begin by recognizing that our perception is skewed by our biases, our feelings, our hopes, our history, our anger, our desires. We also recognize that our perception is skewed by our brain which takes shortcuts to reach conclusions more easily and more quickly. We begin, then, by seeking to understand how our ego affects our understanding. A fearless inventory of our beliefs and of the beliefs of our peer group is a place to start. Add to that inventories of our failures, our parents' beliefs, and our prejudices, and we will have begun to gain a clearer vision of the world as it is, not as we would have it be. Without the recognition that we have a problem, we cannot begin to be open to accepting truth when it challenges us to new insights and new ways of being. Unfortunately, because our perception is automatically and unconsciously sorted by the brain on the basis of our personal experience and spirituality, learning to know what we do not know can be a challenging, if not an impossible, task. The place to begin is the recognition that we need help.

(2) In a culture not based on honesty and tolerance, we need to find a group where our perceptions can be tested in a way that does not threaten us personally. This is why in my own ministry I found a support group to be extremely important. This is why good leaders in business work in teams. We need a group that will help us distinguish a fact from a belief or an opinion, a group that does not attack us for our ideas. We need a group in which there is a culture of fact-finding in order to build an idea that is larger than any individual's position. We need a group that understands that truth and vision may require many different perspectives. We need a group that is grounded in facts while abounding in disagreements, but united in the common goal of reaching truthful insights and making sound decisions. Living in a culture formed by competition and status, to discover truth we need a group where the culture is formed by honesty, love, and tolerance.

(3) As we live into the reality that we do not know all we think we know, and that in order to gain greater objectivity and insight we need help, we will discover that listening is an essential tool for the journey toward

truth. When we listen carefully, seeking to understand the other's position rather than looking for flaws in the other's ideas, we may have to modify our own understanding. This ability requires a strong person; one who is able to be influenced by others while also being able to influence others.

(4) Finally, a diversity of voices that we listen to and interact with is essential. Recognizing we are biased and cannot know truth by our own efforts alone and building a group to introduce other options and inspire insight is only the beginning point in the pursuit for truth. Even with these efforts we are still confined by our particular culture. I think about my own life and recognize those moments when I grew emotionally and intellectually were those times I was involved with a group from a different culture: the interracial group when I was in high school; living and working in West Chicago the summer before race riots burned much of the neighborhood; living and working in Santo Domingo the summer after the revolution; my small group of members of A.A. and my continued involvement with the Fellowship; living and working ten years in a working-class community; and more. We cannot overestimate the importance of cross-cultural experiences. Among other gains, they help us realize that in fact there is much we do not know.

Perhaps truth is best approached and captured as a process rather than as a destination. This understanding of truth as truth-seeking is not new. In many ways the scientific method is similar. The great physicist Edwin Hubble, speaking at Caltech's commencement in 1938, said a scientist has "a healthy skepticism, suspended judgement, and disciplined imagination"—not only about other people's ideas but also about his or her own. The scientist has an experimental mind, not a litigious one.[10] Further, such truth-seeking is the effort not of a single person but of a group of people—the bigger the better—who pursue ideas with curiosity, inquisitiveness, openness, and discipline. Scientists retest, or validate, what is already known, and build upon the last discovery. They observe the world with an open mind, gathering facts and testing predictions and expectations against them. But even the best conclusion is not seen as completely settled. John Wheeler, the eminent American theoretical physicist, described this unending pursuit of truth with this famous quote, "We live on an island surrounded by a sea of ignorance. As the island of our knowledge grows, so does the shore of our ignorance."[11] All knowledge is just probable knowl-

10. Gawande, "Mistrust of Science," para. 2.
11. Horgan, "Do Our Questions Create the World?"

edge. A contradictory piece of evidence can always emerge. As Hubble said, "The scientist explains the world by successive approximations."[12]

Kahneman and Tversky offer an illustration in the way they worked. They are described by many as dramatically different personalities. Amos Tversky was one of the most brilliant minds in the university, always believing he was right; he attacked any argument he felt was illogical. Danny Kahneman was always sure he was wrong; if an idea seemed illogical, he asked what truth might be found in it. Tversky was a late-night person, the life of every party, loose and informal, tone-deaf but loved to sing Hebrew folk songs. Kahneman was a morning person. He didn't go to parties, always seemed formal, and never sang. He was a pessimist and took everything seriously. Eager to please, he was so susceptible to criticism that a simple remark could send him into severe self-doubt. Tversky was an optimist and thought pessimism was stupid. He liked to turn things into a joke. He could not understand why anyone would be eager to please. Not surprisingly, Danny Kahneman was seen as a high-maintenance person, while Amos Tversky seemed to be the last person to put up with a high-maintenance person. Even their offices were dramatically different. Amos Tversky's office was extremely clean—no papers or books on his desk, nothing more than a pencil. Kahneman's office was a huge mess with books left open where he had stopped reading, papers in a variety of places, and scraps of paper with important notes scattered over the desk.

Both were supremely interested in how people functioned in unemotional mode. Both were focused on what they and fellow scientists thought they knew but in fact did not know. They had a style of working in which they just talked to each other—hour after hour after hour, often hollering at each other, more often laughing, back and forth, switching between Hebrew and English. Their collaboration was so complete that neither of them felt comfortable taking the credit as the head author. On their first article to decide whose name was to appear first, they flipped a coin. In subsequent articles, they alternated whose name was first.

Their style, and I suggest the reason for their breakthrough new insights, reflects in minuscule the approach we have just described as the truth-seeking process in the Twelve-Step groups. (1) Their focus was on knowing what they did not know, accepting the carefully tested conclusions, and then building on those insights to know more that we do not presently know. (2) They worked in a culture where new ideas were welcomed. (3)

12. Gawande, "Mistrust of Science," para. 3.

Because they were such different personalities, the time they spent in dialogue led to the examination of many different perspectives. (4) They took the time necessary to sort through the many possibilities. They went over each sentence again and again. A sentence, or at most a paragraph, might be the complete work for a day.

Likewise, as we seek to define a pragmatic spirituality, we recognize that truth is both essential and constantly evolving. Each meeting, each new experience, brings new insights and understanding, as those who have attended years of A.A. meetings will affirm. That truth is constantly evolving does not imply total relativity. When people hold differing beliefs, one will be closer to reality, but to discover which requires much conversation and careful listening. Each new insight builds on previous insights and positions. There is a reality we seek to know, and seeking requires humility.

At the center of truth-seeking is dialogue. To grow in true wisdom and knowledge requires a seeking and an exchange, ideally in a culture that supports truth-telling with tolerance. To grow in true wisdom and knowledge requires listening as well as putting thoughts together as conclusions. It requires testing hypotheses and revising beliefs. This process is most productive when the community is truly diverse, with voices from a multitude of cultures, genders, classes, races, and ages. To recognize we cannot find truth alone, that truth depends on dialogue, is to recognize that the source of authority is in one's relationships.

When Jesus said, "I am the truth," (John 14:16) perhaps he did not mean he knew all there is to know about ethics and theology; perhaps he meant that being in relationship with a loving, accepting, and tolerant person is the way to understanding.

CHAPTER 6

Community as Transformative Power

Meetings

In October 2012, hurricane Sandy hit New York City and surrounding areas, inflicting incredible damage. The week before Sandy made landfall, the World Service meeting of Alcoholics Anonymous was held in Rye, New York. International delegates from around the world had gathered to work and learn from each other. Their meeting concluded on Friday, but many stayed to observe the quarterly meeting of the trustees of the General Service Board, which convened that Saturday, Sunday, and Monday, before Sandy hit. Due to the coming storm we cancelled Monday's meeting, instead choosing to meet on Sunday evening. While some of the trustees were able to leave on Monday morning, many of the international delegates and about half of the trustees were stuck in the Hilton Hotel in Rye when Sandy hit. They were left without power or water.

The crews that were working to repair the electrical damage in the area also moved into the darkened hotel. The second night after two rigorous, long days, working under extremely difficult conditions, one of the workers was particularly hostile—toward the hotel management, toward other workers, and toward those trustees and delegates who were stranded in the hotel. In his tirade he asked, "What the hell are you doing here anyway?" Someone explained who they were and that they were stranded until flights could be resumed. "God," he said, "I could use a meeting right now!" Yes, he was also a member of A.A. So candles were found, a few flashlights still worked, a Big Book was brought out, and a meeting was held there in the darkened lobby of the hotel. An hour later the worker was calm and pleasant, though still fatigued. The meeting was transformative.

As discussed earlier, when the Big Book was first published in 1939, regular group meetings were not viewed as an essential part of the program. As membership grew, partly as a result of the book's publication, very quickly groups were seen as essential for the movement. The Twelve Traditions developed later embody this recognition, providing structure for the Fellowship.

Much of the power of A.A. comes from the quality of the community in its meetings. What is it about these meetings that makes them powerful enough to transform a person's life? What is it about these meetings that makes it possible for someone to stop drinking? How are meetings able to do what personal efforts, strong will, psychologists, and righteous/religious persons are unable to do?

I do not pretend to give an adequate explanation. I recognize this process of transformation that comes through gathering and sharing is a mystery beyond final analysis. I also know that millions of alcoholics have found a new, healthy, productive, and joyful life by gathering in groups and sharing their personal stories. I see members' lives change; I see the personal movement from being self-absorbed to becoming a highly reliable servant to other suffering alcoholics. And I recognize this process—a mystery beyond final analysis—is experienced by millions. What is it about meetings that makes the impossible possible for millions of alcoholics?

Groups

Before we explore this question further, I turn to some insights about groups that come from sociology, current business theory, and recent biblical scholarship.

Every group, every institution—a football team, a business, a Habitat for Humanity group, a church, a Twelve-Step group, a nation—has an outer aspect—the visible organization, the members, the buildings possessed by the group, etc.—and an inner aspect—the unseen values, dreams, and mores of the people involved, both past and present. This inner nature is not some separate entity, but is an invisible aspect of the material organization. In business theory this inner, invisible aspect is called the "culture." Perhaps it is because I am an ordained minister, but I prefer the word "spirit." In this book I use "culture" and "spirit" interchangeably. Whichever word we use, the spirit, the culture of a group or an organization is an invisible reality that exists as an integral part of the organization.

Significantly, this spirit, this culture of an organization, is more than a personification of certain aspects of the group or institution; it is a strong power that influences the individuals who are members of the group. In other words, terms like "mob spirit" or "team spirit" or *"esprit de corps"* describe realities that come into existence when a mob or a team forms, causing people to act in ways they never believed themselves capable of acting alone. If you have played team sports, you know that at times the team was up, and each member performed better; and at times the team was down, and the players made multiple errors in judgment and performance. The job of a coach is not only to help players improve their skills and to develop strategy for the game; it is also to nurture a positive team spirit. You have also probably been at one time or another in a group of complaining people. How easy it is in such an environment to become negative. Or conversely, being part of a group that works hard at a task will result in your working harder than you usually do. Groups have a power, an invisible reality, that exerts great influence on the members and that is a powerful guiding force for the organization. Why do lawyers tend to wear suits while IT workers wear T-shirts or turtlenecks? Why do people apologize when they swear in front of clergy? Why is success equated with a higher salary? The spirits of institutions and the spirit of our society govern dress, social class, life expectation, even the choice of a marriage partner. Every organization—formal or informal, large or small—contains a spirit, a culture.

Because the institution usually antedates and outlasts the members, it develops and imposes a set of traditions, expectations, beliefs, and values on everyone in the group. Usually unspoken, unacknowledged, and even unconscious, this invisible network of influences and standards constrains behavior far more than any printed set of rules could ever do. Contemporary business theory seeks to address the culture of a company through mission and vision statements combined with lists of values. Too often, unfortunately, these statements do not align with the germane essence of the culture that actually guides the workers. Before management can modify the spirit of a corporation, they must truly understand the actual values and practices that make up the culture. It is easy to underestimate the strength of this invisible guiding power and seek to impose actions and an alternative culture; it rarely works.

Twelve Steps to Religionless Spirituality

I have a friend, a college student, who took a summer job with a construction crew. Anxious to be seen as an outstanding worker by his supervisor, he arrived early, worked hard, took only the ten minutes allowed for break, and even worked into lunch. At this point one of the older workmen took him aside and instructed him on worker's expectations. "We don't over-do. If break takes fifteen or twenty minutes, that's OK. Lunch often takes one and a half hours. If we are at a stopping point, we may quit a little early. Just wanted you to know how we do it around here." My friend understood that if he wanted to work with these men, he would have to learn to do it their way.

My secretary at Trinity Church, Buffalo, where I served as Rector, would come into my office from time to time to announce, "Ward, there are four ways to accomplish what you want to do: there's a right way, a wrong way, your way, and the Trinity way. I suggest this time we follow the Trinity way." That was always helpful advice.

The origin of a group culture or spirit eludes easy, formulaic explanation. It is not likely to evolve from imposed direction, but rather it is a function of the group's shared values which then filter who will become part of the group.

Remarkably, the spirit of Alcoholics Anonymous, defined by a set of spiritual principles, has remained consistent and powerful since its founding. The Preamble, the Steps, the Traditions, and "How it Works," which are read at most meetings, define and reinforce the spirit of acceptance, surrender, inclusion, honesty, unity, humility, and purpose that guides the members. The organizational structure is decentralized; this spirit, not trustees or managers, guides A.A.

In my experience, in a healthy A.A. group there is a spirit of acceptance, of accountability, of truth, of gratitude, of love. That spirit, that culture, is in fact a power greater than any of the individual members. I suggest it is that spirit that is able to do what personal efforts, strong will, psychologists, and the righteous/religious are unable to do. It is that spirit that makes the impossible possible. Members of A.A. know this; they have experienced it. Members of other groups—a business, a sports team, a school, a neighborhood, a church—also experience the power present in the spirit, the culture of the groups to which they belong. Many, perhaps most, members of A.A. understand this spirit as the Spirit of God; atheists and agnostics in A.A. understand it as the *esprit de corps*. But both believers and nonbelievers experience this spirit as a power greater than themselves that makes change and a new life possible for them.

We tend to think of spirituality as an individual activity. We tend to associate spiritual practice with meditation, prayer, silent retreats, walking in the woods, and the like—getting away from it all to find and be in touch with God. Even church, which involves a gathering of people, may seem to many like an individual experience: people don't speak to each other, don't know one another, and expect the sermon to be inspiring and the music to be uplifting. While individual spiritual practices are important, spirituality involves much more than the individual. The culture of one's place of employment, the quality of family life, the neighborhood spirit (or lack thereof), and the groups one is part of all influence a person's spirituality. As discussed in the earlier chapter on spirituality, one's activities, one's spiritual practices, one's history, what one reads or watches, and the groups one participates in all become woven together in the individual's spirit—for better or for worse. In our contemporary American perspective, which focuses on the individual, the ability of groups to have major influence over our spirituality is largely neglected. For example, to work for racial justice we must be aware of the history of racism, the contemporary culture, hate groups, and hate literature in order to make progress. Only within this larger context can progress be made.

Groups are powerful influences on one's spiritual development; it is important to be intentional about the groups in which we participate. It is also important that we support the positive aspects of these groups.

Communities

In July 1995, a scorching heat wave hit Chicago, killing 739 people (about seven times as many as died in Hurricane Sandy). Soon after the heat abated, social scientists began to look for patterns behind the deaths. Some results were unsurprising, like having a working air conditioner was a lifesaver. Also, as one would expect, the geography of heat wave mortality was consistent with the city's geography of segregation and inequality. Eight of the ten communities with the highest death rates were virtually all African American with pockets of concentrated poverty and violent crime. Surprisingly, however, three of the ten neighborhoods with the lowest death rates were also poor, violent, and predominantly African American. One example stood out: two adjacent neighborhoods on the South Side

of Chicago, both 99 percent African American, both with similar propor-
tions of elderly residents, both with high rates of poverty, unemployment,
and violent crime. One (Englewood) had thirty-three deaths per 100,000
which was one of the highest rates; the other (Auburn Gresham) had only
three deaths per 100,000, making it safer than many of the most affluent
neighborhoods on the North Side.[1]

What caused this difference? Many studies have explored this in an effort to understand the predictors of outcomes. With climate change we are
expecting more such disasters, and we need to know how to survive. The
research concluded that while government services and infrastructure had
a role to play, the primary difference lay in the quality of community—good
social networks and connections. While demographically similar, the two
neighborhoods turned out to be differentiated by those aspects of community that bring people into contact with friends and neighbors.

Between 1960 and 1990, Englewood (the neighborhood with the high
mortality rate) lost 50 percent of its residents and most of its commercial
outlets.[2] Without shops, restaurants, and other community organizations,
the people of Englewood no longer knew the people across the street. The
elderly were apprehensive about leaving their homes. By contrast, the other
neighborhood experienced no population loss during that same period. In
1995, residents walked to diners and grocery stores; they knew their neighbors; they participated in block clubs and church groups. During the heat
wave, they knew who was alone, who was elderly, who was sick; and they
checked on them. That was the difference—the quality of community—and
it saved lives. In fact, in follow-up studies, researchers discovered that in
1990 life expectancy in Englewood was five years lower than in the Auburn
Gresham neighborhood.[3]

If the quality of life within a community is a primary factor in the
emotional, spiritual, and physical health of the individuals within the
neighborhood, can it work the other way around? Can individuals build
a group that will transform their neighborhood? The answer is yes, but it
takes effort and time. This power of the group is one of the most important
tools that is emerging in areas and neighborhoods of extreme poverty and
lack of services. The South Bronx Churches provide an example I know
personally.

1. Klinenberg, "Adaptation," paras. 1 and 2.
2. Klinenberg, "Adaptation," para. 26.
3. Klinenberg, "Adaptation," para. 27.

The South Bronx in New York City has for decades struggled with poverty, poor education, health problems, drug dealers, alcohol abuse, and crime. It was one of the poorest neighborhoods, not only in New York City, but in the entire United States. Government programs, well-meaning volunteers, and social service agencies have had little effect in bringing improved conditions. Then in 1986, an elderly woman waiting for a train was killed in an apparent attempted robbery in a subway station. Many had been complaining for years regarding safety in the area—street lights that did not work, drug dealers who sold with impunity, no street signs, garbage left uncollected. By and large, religious institutions were the only social agencies remaining in the neighborhood; so local pastors and lay leaders from churches, synagogues, and mosques gathered. Following the example of other poorer neighborhoods in the city, they decided they must organize to bring change to their neighborhood. They developed core groups; they did one-on-one interviews throughout the community and developed issue lists; they raised money. In 1987, they hired an organizer and became the South Bronx Churches (SBC) organization.

They reached out to other organizations—East Brooklyn Churches, Harlem Congregations for Community Improvement—and through large community meetings decided where to begin. They needed success, so they began small. A thousand people turned out as they made their demand of the Metropolitan Transit Authority to clean and light subway stations—they got results. They sent volunteers into the grocery stores, dressed in white coats, carrying clip boards, to make notes on the poor quality of the produce—even though the volunteers were not connected with any government agency, the improvements were dramatic. They worked with the police, demanding and getting better law enforcement.

As they gained strength, they turned to the need for quality housing. In the 1980s, as the crack cocaine epidemic spread through the South Bronx, there was a major exodus. Landlords could not afford to pay the taxes on their buildings. Arson filled the need to liquidate assets. The result was block after block of abandoned, burned-out buildings. SBC negotiated with the city to donate the land; they developed financial resources through banks without federal and state aid; and they negotiated with contractors to build modest single-family homes and apartments. From 1990 to 1995 they built and sold over 1,000 homes. There have been almost no foreclosures, and abandoned lots have become thriving communities.

Then they took up the problems of education. Working with the New York City Department of Education (DOE), in 1993 they launched the Bronx Leadership Academy. In 1996, it graduated its first class with a 90 percent graduation rate and with 85 percent of the graduates being admitted to college. They have since opened another Leadership Academy and in 2010—jointly with the DOE—they opened the Mott Haven Campus public high school, a state-of-the-art facility that serves 2,200 students and offers a broad range of community services. More recently, with other metro organizations they successfully pushed the DOE to invest $22 million in more services for special needs students, and to establish a team to fix their broken special education data system.

Alone as individuals the people of the South Bronx were no more able to improve their living conditions than alcoholics by their own efforts are able to stop drinking. But together they have the power to collaborate with or to confront powerful institutions in the governmental and private sectors. Multiracial, multicultural, multidenominational, and multifaith, they are able to affirm their basic identity as human beings who care about each other and about their neighborhood. Such community organizations are pragmatic; have agendas set by the members, not the leaders; are non-partisan, not favoring or supporting any party; and focus only on those issues and strategies that enrich their communities directly. Each successive outcome yields dignity and greater opportunity, and strengthens the core values of the group. Such is the transformative power of community to bring dignity to the individual and transformation to the neighborhood. [4]

The transformative power of community can be experienced in a group like A.A., in a neighborhood where the quality of life is supportive, or in an organized group like SBC. When there is a strong, positive community, people's lives are strengthened, renewed, and empowered.

Mutuality

On Saturday, May 11, 1935, after years of struggling with alcoholism, having found a fragile sobriety as a result of a religious experience while hospitalized for this disease, Bill W. was sitting in a hotel lobby in Akron, Ohio, at the end of an unsuccessful business encounter. Across from where he sat was the bar, filled with people who seemed to be happily enjoying

4. For more information, see www.sbc-iaf.org. and www.industrialareasfoundation. org.

themselves. He thought about his lost proxy fight and the reality that he had no job. He thought about Mother's Day and how his wife would be disappointed that he was not with her in New York.

"God," he thought, "I am going to get drunk." He panicked. Never before had he panicked at the thought of a drink. An idea arose out of his recent experiences, "I need another alcoholic."

At the other end of the lobby was a church directory. He needed someone like those he knew from the Oxford Group meeting at Calvary Episcopal Church in New York. He picked out the name of the Episcopal priest, The Rev. Walter Tunks. Thus began a series of calls that resulted in his connection with Mrs. Henrietta Seiberling. He began, "I'm from the Oxford Group, and I'm a rum hound from New York." Mrs. Seiberling, a committed member of the Oxford Group, had spent the last two years trying to sober up her close friend's husband, a prominent surgeon, Dr. Bob S. She invited Bill to come to her home. She arranged for the two of them to meet. Instead of preaching at Dr. Bob or trying to tell him the medical advice he had learned, Bill began by sharing the tale of his experiences with alcohol—the hopes, the promises, and the failures of both. In *Alcoholics Anonymous Comes of Age*, Bill explains why this conversation was different—why, after his earlier failures this meeting had worked:

> You see, our talk was a completely mutual thing . . . I knew that I needed this alcoholic as much as he needed me. *This was it.* And this mutual give-and-take is at the very heart of all of A.A.'s Twelfth Step work today. The final missing link was located right there in my first talk with Dr. Bob.[5]

Mutuality is the key—Bill needed Dr. Bob as much as Dr. Bob needed him. Where there is mutuality, true mutuality, the bond is greater, the commitment is stronger, the self-focus is diminished, and the possibility for growth and service is enhanced.

Mutuality may come from a variety of shared experiences or shared purposes. Groups can develop strong mutual relationships when they pursue a common task. Military companies which share both the risk of physical harm and commitment to a tactical goal become very close. Athletic teams may become bound together by their common goals. People who work together on projects, like building a home through Habitat for Humanity, are strengthened by the closeness they feel with the group. But

---

5. Bill W., *Alcoholics Anonymous Comes of Age*, 70 (italics original).

for groups to become truly mutual, almost always the foundation is built on the sharing of personal suffering.

The Spanish philosopher Miguel de Unamuno said it this way:

> . . . spiritual love is born of sorrow. . . . For [people] love one another with a spiritual love only when they have suffered the same sorrow together, when through long days they have ploughed the stony ground buried beneath the common yoke of a common grief. It is then that they know one another and feel one another, and feel with one another in their common anguish, and thus they pity one another and love one another.[6]

A favorite story about mutuality:

> A farmer had some puppies he needed to sell. He painted a sign advertising the four pups and set about nailing it to a post on the edge of his yard. As he was driving the last nail into the post, he felt a tug on his overalls. He looked down into the eyes of a little boy.
>
> "Mister," he said, "I want to buy one of your puppies."
>
> "Well," said the farmer, as he rubbed the sweat off the back of his neck, "these puppies come from fine parents and cost a good deal of money."
>
> The boy dropped his head for a moment. Then reaching deep into his pocket, he pulled out a handful of change and held it up to the farmer.
>
> "I've got thirty-nine cents. Is that enough to take a look?"
>
> "Sure," said the farmer. And with that he let out a whistle. "Here, Dolly!" he called.
>
> Out from the doghouse and down the ramp ran Dolly followed by four little balls of fur.
>
> The little boy pressed his face against the chain-link fence. His eyes danced with delight. As the dogs made their way to the fence, the little boy noticed something else stirring inside the doghouse.
>
> Slowly another little ball appeared, this one noticeably smaller. Down the ramp it slid. Then in a somewhat awkward manner, the little pup began hobbling toward the others, doing its best to catch up.
>
> "I want that one," the little boy said, pointing to the runt.
>
> The farmer knelt down at the boy's side and said, "Son, you don't want that puppy. He will never be able to run and play with you like these other dogs would."

6. Unamuno, *Tragic Sense of Life*, 135–36.

With that the little boy stepped back from the fence, reached down, and began rolling up one leg of his trousers. In doing so he revealed a steel brace running down both sides of this leg attaching itself to a specially made shoe.

Looking back up at the farmer, he said, "You see, sir, I don't run too well myself, and he will need someone who understands."

With tears in his eyes, the farmer reached down and picked up the little pup. Holding it carefully, he handed it to the little boy.

"How much?" asked the little boy.

"No charge," answered the farmer, "there is no charge for love." [7]

Mutuality is a key factor in the development of strong communities, but it is not easy. It requires a strong person to develop mutual relationships. Mutuality requires the ability to listen carefully to the other, to be open to changing one's own opinion or position, and to still maintain a sense of self, to still maintain one's own identity and responsibility. Mutuality means one can be affected by others as well as being able to affect others. Mutuality is the building block of cooperative communities that, like A.A., can change our world.

Mary was a fine athlete in high school—a record holder on the swim team and a star on the volleyball team. In her school it was the practice that the coach appointed the captain of the teams. Mary had served as captain of the volleyball team, but on a day she was absent from school, the coach appointed Jane to be captain of the swim team. Mary was angry.

"Jane doesn't hold a single record," she yelled at me. "She thinks she is so good, but she really does not train or work hard enough. There is no reason she should be captain. She never congratulated me when I was appointed volleyball team captain; I won't congratulate her."

I asked her, "Do you think that will help the team?"

She gave me a hard look and stalked out of the room.

The next day I saw Mary as she was walking home from school. "Well," she said, "I congratulated Jane. I hope you are happy. I still don't think she deserves to be captain, but I want the team to get along. That is important."

It takes a big person to swallow pride and return kindness for rudeness and insult. It takes a strong person to accept criticism without becoming defensive. It takes this kind of strength to nurture cooperative communities.

The concept of surrender applies here. Surrender of self to become a part of the greater whole involves the recognition that the whole is more

7. Kurtz and Ketcham, *Experiencing Spirituality,* 92–94.

powerful and a higher good than any individual. At first, one is attracted to the group because it provides hope that life can be better. But as life in the group progresses and trust begins to emerge, one must surrender personal agendas and desires in favor of the overall unity of the group. Hope evolves to trust, which evolves to surrender, which evolves to faith. It requires letting go, detachment, which represents a major transformation. Now we see why surrender is such an important spiritual principle. It is out of this surrender that new life emerges, a new life built on mutual relationships and shared service. To be able to let go of control and be led by the concerns of the group is not weakness but is a sign of strength. Mutual relationships involve not the bargained give-and-take of cooperation; rather, mutual relationships involve genuine giving, with the result that one receives more than they thought imaginable—they are always gifts, not contractual agreements. It may seem counterintuitive, but the skill of surrendering, listening, and opening one's mind and heart in mutuality, particularly in the setting of community, can yield the fiercest clarity, determination, and effectiveness. When Jesus said the meek shall inherit the earth (Matt 5:5), I do not believe he meant we should be doormats; I believe he meant those who are strong enough to sacrifice themselves for others, those who are able to swallow pride in order to encourage mutual relationships and nurture collaborative communities; these will transform the earth.

Communities of Compassion

I have a friend who shares a somewhat different story. She was struggling with an alcoholic husband, her second; she was angry, depressed, and feeling like a total failure. A friend invited her to come be part of a small group that met weekly at the friend's church. This small group program consisted of a presentation by the minister, followed by the group, which met without the minister to discuss how they saw the content of the presentation in relation to their lives. While no one was asked to share their personal story, the group provided an opportunity to share what was happening to a person— painful or joyful. My friend began to share some of what was happening in her home. She tells me she has no memory of any of the presentations, but she does remember that the group truly loved and cared for her. She told me they would express their support and concern, and she would think, "If you only knew. . . ." Then a tragic event occurred—the death of her stepson. The next morning members of the group appeared at her home with crab cakes, and they listened. Slowly she came to accept that she must be lovable since they clearly loved and cared for her. Slowly she came to accept that she was worth fixing and went to a counselor. The counselor was wise; she asked my friend to take an inventory of her own drinking. The next week my friend came to the counselor with the realization that she too had a drinking problem. After a thirty-day treatment in a residential program, she began attending A.A. and continues to do so at present. Having been loved into health by the small group at church, she was able to make the choice to seek greater health. Today she now loves others into health and continues her spiritual journey on the road to a happy destiny.

I believe that nurturing such loving communities is what Jesus was primarily about. When one considers what Jesus actually did in the few years of his public ministry, it does not seem earth-transforming. He healed a few people, he provided food for a large crowd on at least one, maybe two, occasions. He taught. He attracted large crowds occasionally. He confronted the power structure. But if his goal was to reform current Jewish practices or to lead a social revolution, one might suggest he failed.

For one thing, he refused to be honored as the Messiah who would lead a revolution. He left in the night when the people were about to make him king (John 6:15). When the crowds were growing larger, he told Peter they needed to go elsewhere (Mark 1:38). Even when he was addressed as "Good Master," he responded that only God is good (Mark 10:17–18). Clearly, collecting large numbers of enthusiastic followers was not his primary concern. It is almost as though he wanted to be anonymous!

When Jesus heard of his friend Lazarus's death, he returned to Bethany to be with Mary and Martha, Lazarus's sisters (John 11:1–44). We easily focus on the miracle of the raising of Lazarus from the dead, but I believe the important part of the story is how Jesus arrived in Bethany. His arrival is summed up in one verse: "Jesus wept" (John 11:35). He did not come unfeeling, self-assured, saying: I'm here now; all is well. He came as a vulnerable person, with empathy, seeing the pain of his friends, weeping with them in their sorrow. The miracle comes from the power of that pain and compassion, not the magic of a supernatural savior.

One other story: this one happened in the region of Tyre and Sidon (Mark 7:24–30). Jesus was taking a little time off, heading north, away from Galilee, toward the beach. A very human Jesus, probably tired, was approached by an insistent Syrian woman of Phoenicia pleading with him to heal her sick daughter. His disparaging remark (in response to her request) about taking the children's bread and casting it to a dog reflects the prejudice of his own culture which formed his attitudes and beliefs. But the woman's insistence compelled him to see that God's compassion was for all, including this gentile's daughter. In healing the daughter, Jesus was able to transcend his culture and its limitations because he was a compassionate listener.

What the record tells us that Jesus actually did is dramatically different from the popular conception of an omnicompetent collector of thousands of satisfied customers. What Jesus did was focus on a small band of followers. That group was radically inclusive, being made up of both women and men, members of the working class, a tax collector who worked for the hated Roman Empire, and a Zealot who violently opposed Roman occupation. He struggled to teach them clearly about the compassionate God and the social and political ramifications of such compassion. They were slow learners, but in the community he formed they experienced that inclusive, healing compassion. Yes, he attracted large crowds, but his focus was on the small group that would be leaders. Jesus' focus was on nurturing a community of compassion as an expression of what life is intended to be. I believe that Christianity spread because such communities are so life-giving.

I would agree with the Jewish theologian Martin Buber that community is God's goal for creation—a healthy, loving, supportive, creative, even challenging community. The biblical story runs from the garden of Eden in Genesis to the new Jerusalem of Revelation. We are headed toward an abundant, inclusive, open, accepting community bathed by the light of divine love. Jesus' teaching on the kingdom of God is best understood as teaching about the quality of life that is known in a community of compassion.

What I have learned from A.A. is that not only is community the goal of human history, it is also the means we have to move toward that goal. There is incredible power in community—at the level of interpersonal relationships, at the civic level, as the church, as an A.A. group; wherever two or three are gathered together in a mutual community, a power is present that transforms human lives and human society. Some identify this power as the love of God.

Community, Identity, and Purpose

Earlier this year I listened to an interview of a young man who had been a member of a gang and who is now working with gang members, helping them become free and lead healthy and productive lives. When asked why people become members of gangs, he responded that there are three things we all seek: identity, community, and purpose. For those without much hope for the future, gangs can provide these. Although I tend to view gangs with a negative bias, I thought this understanding of why groups are important was insightful and helpful.

Identity, community, and purpose are fundamental human, spiritual needs and are closely tied together. To be part of a community requires a sense of identity so one knows who they are and who they are not and if they belong to this particular group. And when one finds a group that fits their identity, their identity will be strengthened by the support from the group that provides a setting where they can accept and embrace who they are.

As we shall explore in the next chapter, sharing stories is instrumental in building the community and strengthening the individual's connection to the group. Sharing one's personal story touches the heart. Spirituality is communicated through story far more than through exposition of factual information. The spirituality of the group strengthens one's identity and the sharing of one's personal story is the means that allows a group to become truly mutual. As the stories are told, the group itself finds its own story. Fred's story of his struggles with alcohol parallels Jane's story and Juanita's story and Amos's story. And the group story emerges as a place that brings healing and new life. And from that story emerges an understanding of the purpose of the group—to reach out to those who are still suffering and need healing and new life.

The process of the story-sharing that occurs when joining a group, finding mutuality, and creating a cohesive community is infused with several elements. There is an investment of time. The giving of that time is a sacrifice of value which strengthens the community outcomes, just as investing time in a friendship strengthens the bond of that friendship. In telling stories, there is a willingness to be truthful, humble, and vulnerable. This risk, when met with acceptance and comfort, results in trust and a further bond with community. And finally, in sharing like stories, one sees how one's individual story parallels that of others, and with that, a unity, a collective, is recognized.

When Fred joined A.A. he found far more than rules to follow. He found a community where he was accepted and supported in his struggle with his disease. He found a welcome from people who truly understood his thoughts and feelings because they too had struggled with alcoholism. Doctor, plumber, homemaker, or teacher—all shared their common history. He also found a new identity, based not on his position or his (poor) performance but on honestly accepting his humanity. To stand up and say, "My name is Fred, and I am an alcoholic," is not an act of shame. Rather it is just the opposite; it is an act of acceptance. As he continued in the Fellowship, Fred developed new understandings about his cunning, baffling, and powerful disease. By becoming a member of A.A., Fred received a new identity; he discovered the strength of mutual support; he found his insights and emotional and spiritual health improving; and he added a new purpose to his life—to support others in the Fellowship of A.A. and to carry the message of hope to the still-suffering alcoholic.

When Juanita joined the South Bronx Churches, she too found much more than a political organization. She became part of a group that shared her anger, resentment, and frustration. She learned to focus those emotions so the result was not silent depression but vocal activism. She learned to commit to the goals the group developed, even when they were not primary goals for her. She went to the training workshops and learned the history and techniques of organizing and how her skills and personality could effectively be part of the effort. She learned the importance of mutual support and that as a member she was not powerless. From powerless depression she moved to resolute action to improve the lives of those around her and in the process grew spiritually and emotionally.

Identity, community, and purpose—central needs for us as human beings. Finding a group that nurtures these three in a healthy manner may be the primary factor in developing spiritual maturity and successful living.

CHAPTER 7

Spirituality and Story

When the great Rabbi Israel Baal Shem-Tov saw misfortune threatening the Jews it was his custom to go into a certain part of the forest to meditate. There he would light a fire, say a special prayer, and the miracle would be accomplished and the misfortune averted.

Later, when his disciple, the celebrated Magid or Mezritch had occasion, for the same reason, to intercede with heaven, he would go to the same place in the forest and say: "Master of the Universe, listen! I do not know how to light the fire, but I am still able to say the prayer." And again, the miracle would be accomplished.

Still later, Rabbi Moshe-Leib of Sasov, in order to save his people once more, would go into the forest and say: "I do not know how to light the fire, I do not know the prayer, but I know the place and this must be sufficient." Once more God produced a miracle to save the Jews.

Then it fell to Rabbi Israel of Rizhyn to overcome misfortune. Sitting in his armchair, his head in his hands, he spoke to God: "I am unable to light the fire and I do not know the prayer; I cannot even find the place in the forest. All I can do is tell the story, and this must be sufficient." And it was sufficient.

God made [human beings] because God loves stories.[1]

ONE'S SPIRITUALITY IS A dynamic, complex, constantly evolving combination of what we perceive, how we feel about our perceptions, and how we respond through the choices we make. These are primarily internal processes. Choices may be seen, though not always. Perception and feelings are

---

1. Wiesel, *Gates of the Forest*, introductory notes.

not observable and are often not even observed by the person who is perceiving and feeling. Even the choices we make may only be vaguely recognized. Spiritual realities are difficult to identify and define. Truth, wisdom,
beauty, fragrance, despair, hope—all these are spiritual matters. We know
and experience them, but because they are intangible, ineffable realities,
we find them difficult to describe in words. We all know the fragrance of a
rose; but how do we describe it with words so one who has not smelled a
rose might understand? We have experiences that a certain person or scene
or sunset or flower is beautiful, but how do we share our experience; how
do we define beauty?

We cannot communicate spirituality with abstract, intellectual terminology. I come closer to communicating about a spiritual reality, like
beauty, by storytelling, by sharing my experience. My wife and I live on the
Tennessee River, which is a two-mile-wide lake where we live. We often
go down to the river bank, usually in the evening, to relax and enjoy the
peace and quiet. There are a few motor boats that pierce the quiet, and
occasionally we hear voices from across the water. If the wind is blowing,
the waves form multiple patterns on the water; if it is calm, the water is like
glass. When the sky is blue, the river reflects and intensifies the color. As the
sun sets, we watch the changing sky—a mixture of clouds, red and orange
sky, bright white rays of sunshine, and gathering darkness. I take her hand;
she lays her head on my shoulder. We do not need to speak. That is beauty.

The difficulty in communicating about spiritual things seems to lie
in the nature of spirituality. To know spiritual things, one must experience
them. The fragrance of a rose, the beauty of a sunset—the only way for
two people to truly understand these is to experience them. Then they may
share their experience. The spiritual, as we have said, are things that cannot
be seen, but which still affect the person. The primary task of words is to
convey ideas; spiritual things must be experienced. And since we continue
to change personally, no one ever experiences the same thing twice, be it a
sunset or a rose.

> The student, who could be any of us, asked his teacher to teach
> him wisdom. The teacher replied, "I would love to teach you wis-
> dom, except wisdom cannot be taught."
>
> The student, saddened by this answer, replied, "Then why
> should I study, why should I seek to learn if I cannot become
> wise?"

"Oh, truly I cannot teach you wisdom, but wisdom can be learned."[2]

An older man, renowned in the rural community for his wisdom was asked by a younger man, "How did you get so wise?"
The old man replied, "It was easy; I have good judgment."
"Then, how did you get good judgment?"
"That's easy," the man replied. "Good judgment comes from experience, and experience comes from having bad judgment."[3]

How do we communicate spiritual realities? How do we share experiences that are private and personal? For many of us one way we seek to share experience is through narrative. Narrative holds the possibility of connecting with the other person's experience. The details of the narrative touch some details in the listener's past and remind them of a similar experience. A good story engages our emotions and invites us to experience the events in the story. Didactic information enters the brain where it may be stored or forgotten. It does not touch the heart; it does not affect our hopes and dreams; it does not change or challenge our values or continue to discomfort us. It is objective information designed to avoid emotions.

Spirituality is communicated through stories. Thus all spiritual disciplines share stories as a means of instruction regarding spirituality. We cannot communicate spirituality with abstract, intellectual terminology. Stories have the capability to touch the heart, the soul, the emotional center of our being. Stories can intrigue us and hook us. We become engaged, gaining one insight, and then another insight at a later time. A story is not limited to a specific event or question but it engages the hearer and provides insights into a multitude of situations.

I did much study of the biblical book of Job, and in 1975 I published a book intended to introduce this classic of biblical literature to the lay reader.[4] Many do not realize that when Job was written, there was no theological problem of unjust suffering. If one suffered from illness or tragedy, the theology of the time declared without exception that suffering was God's punishment for unjust and immoral actions. My thesis: Job was not written to explain unjust suffering, to defend the ways of God. Rather Job was written to defend the sufferer from unjust accusations.

2. Kurtz and Ketcham, *Experiencing Spirituality*, 2.

3. Kurtz and Ketcham, *Experiencing Spirituality*, 288.

4. Ewing, *Job*.

The entire book is a story. Job is the morally perfect man, and yet Job suffers great loss and sorrow. His wealth is taken from him; his sons and daughters die when the house they are in is destroyed by a fierce wind; his servants, with few exceptions, also die; and Job is afflicted with sores that cover his body, and an unsympathetic wife. Three friends come to comfort Job, and the story is dominated by the interaction of Job and his would-be comforters.

Job begins, expressing his great pain, by cursing the day he was born. Job's "friends," caught in the accepted theology of the day (that you suffer because you are being punished for wrongdoing), react by advising Job to repent of whatever wrong he has committed, receive God's forgiveness, and be restored to health and prosperity. They are exhibit A of the damage religious people do when they are certain they know the truth. When Job refuses to repent, they declare more and more vehemently their "correct" theological understanding. Slowly they move from comforters to aggressive, hostile accusers. To support their beliefs, they falsely accuse Job of sin. Job defends himself; he experiences God as absent and uncaring; he sees God as enemy. Finally, in a speech that expresses the highest ethical insight in all of Scripture, he makes his case. Totally alienated, he confronts God, demanding explanation. In the dramatic conclusion, God appears to Job out of a whirlwind, but gives no explanation. Job kneels before the divine revelation, reconciled: "I heard of you by the hearing of the ear, but now my eyes see you"(Job 42:5). While the divine voice is silent regarding unjust suffering, it is clear (just in case we might miss the point of the book) in condemning the three comforters: "You have not spoken of me what is right as my servant Job has" (Job 42:7–8).

This story so dramatically refuted the equation of suffering and punishment that ever since we have sought solutions to the problem of reconciling belief in a loving and just God in the face of unjust suffering. Ironically, many, if not most, popular commentators seek a solution to this problem of unjust suffering in the book of Job!

This story became an important part of my spiritual development. My book was published in the summer of 1975; that fall I moved to Louisville where I became involved with Alcoholics Anonymous. I believe the story of Job opened my eyes to see many of the dynamics present in the disease of alcoholism. Friends and family of alcoholics begin by giving advice based on their rational understanding. "Why do you have to have so many drinks? Just have one or two." "If you can't handle alcohol, just stop."

"We can't spend all this money on booze and pay our bills." And of course this advice is worthless, as the disease of alcoholism renders the alcoholic incapable of making such choices. As the disease progresses, the friends and family progress to accusations, suspicion, anger, and out-of-control attempts to control. The alcoholic also progresses, not only through the physical stages of the illness, but also through self-defense to emotional roller coasters toward alienation and despair. The alcoholic may also experience God as absent and as enemy.

I do not believe the author of Job was writing about alcoholism. But in narrating the dynamics of what happens between friends when advice becomes unjust judgment, he described what I was beginning to see in the families in my congregation, where cunning, baffling, and powerful alcohol was destroying lives. Would I have seen alcoholism as a disease if I had not done the work on Job? I don't know; I would hope so. But Job helped prepare me to see what previously I had rationalized and denied.

This is the power of story. A story is not limited to a specific event or question, but it engages the hearer and provides insights into a multitude of situations. I am convinced that a philosophical paper stating that some very good people suffer and that such suffering seems unjust would never have had the impact of the book of Job. Certainly it would never touch anyone emotionally. Without question, such papers had little impact on me.

A good story engages our emotions and may function to entertain us, but beyond the entertainment, much of the inherent appeal of narrative may lie in its ability to abstract and simulate social experience. Stories provide condensed accounts of fundamental social dynamics in human life, and they do so in a way that engages our emotions. Stories teach us how to be human. This is why it is so important to read stories to children.

The Language of the Heart

Change comes when we have been touched emotionally. Theology, doctrine, and intellectual arguments do not touch us emotionally; we are touched emotionally through actions and stories. This, of course, is why I cannot do Twelve-Step calls, even when I have been involved, as in the auto accident described earlier. I have a lot of information about alcoholism, about intervention and treatment, and about Alcoholics Anonymous. Information, however, is a poor vehicle for transmitting hope. Hope is fundamentally a spiritual reality, and we cannot communicate spirituality with abstract, intellectual terminology. We need to touch the heart, the soul, the emotional center of one's being.

In order to communicate hope, one needs to share a story, a story of despair and new life, a story with which a hopeless person can identify. Hope is born when the hopeless alcoholic hears their story on another's lips, and the other is sober, happy, joyous, and free. Hope is born when the drunk discovers that they are not alone. A.A. surrounds them with people who understand. Abstract intellectual understandings cannot connect in the same way. Stories are the way we share experience and spirituality.

We understand this. Change does not come because we have been convinced intellectually that something is the right thing to do. How many times have I heard from my dentist about the importance of flossing my teeth? I believe it is important. I believe it will help prevent dental problems. I just don't floss when I brush my teeth. Intellectual assent does not motivate action. Motivation emerges from a deeper level of values and emotion.

For those caught in the chaos of addiction, hope is the most important tool to encourage them to get help. The way hope is communicated is by one (now sober) drunk sharing their story with another. As noted earlier, because I am not able to do this, I developed a different way. When I get a call from someone that a family member has just been arrested with his third DWI and may lose his driver's license, I call a friend who is an active member in A.A. and together we go visit the family. I talk with the sober member and my friend talks with the drinker. I share information about the disease of alcoholism and the importance of family members getting help. My friend shares her story with the drunk, helping him accept that he has a disease, that he is not alone, and that there is a solution. These interventions have generally proved to be effective.

At the heart of Twelve-Step spirituality is the sharing of personal stories because spirituality is communicated most effectively through story. This storytelling is often referred to as the "language of the heart;" it has power that connects and changes lives. Abstract intellectual understandings cannot connect in the same way. Stories are the way we share experience, emotion, and spirituality.

As Bill W. tells the story of his own intervention by Ebby T., he had learned from Dr. Silkworth (known as the "little doctor who loved drunks") that he suffered from an "infernal malady." After months of working to assist Bill, Dr. Silkworth told him the difficult truth. In Bill's words:

He found the courage gently but frankly to tell us (Bill and his wife Lois) the whole truth: Neither mine nor his nor any other resources he knew could stop my drinking; I would have to be locked up or suffer brain damage or death within perhaps a year.

He spoke in the name of science, which I deeply respected, and by science I seemed condemned.

I was in precisely this state of inner collapse when, in November of 1934, I was visited by Ebby. He was an old friend, an alcoholic, and my sponsor-to-be. Why was it that he could communicate with me in areas that not even Dr. Silkworth could touch?

Well, first of all, I already knew that he himself was a hopeless case—just like me. Earlier that year, I had heard that he, too, was a candidate for the lockup. Yet here he was, sober and free. And his powers of communication now were such that he could convince me in minutes that he really felt he had been released from his drinking compulsion. He represented something very different from a mere jittery ride on the water-wagon. And so he brought me a kind of communication and evidence that even Dr. Silkworth could not give. Here was *one drunk talking to another*. Here was hope indeed.

Ebby told me his story, carefully detailing his drinking experiences of recent years. Thus he drew me still closer to him. I knew beyond doubt that he had lived in that strange and hopeless world where I still was . . . This fact established his identification with me. At length, our channel of communication was wide open, and I was ready for his message.

None of Ebby's ideas were really new. I'd heard them all before . . . But coming over his powerful transmission line, they were not at all what in other circumstances I would have regarded as conventional cliches for good church behavior. They appeared to me as living truths *which might liberate me as they had liberated him.*[5]

Sharing one's story is, of course, central in open meetings. It is the heart of A.A. spirituality. But surprisingly, it became so somewhat circuitously. As friends and colleagues of Bill were reading the drafts of the first edition of the Big Book, the question arose regarding how to end the book. Most of the endings seemed preachy. Dr. Silkworth was asked to write a piece on the nature of addiction, but then it was decided to place that in the front as a preface. Finally it was decided what was needed were testimonials, stories that would show that this program really worked. Sharing one's

---

5. Bill W., *Language of the Heart*, 244–45 (italics original).

story had already become the normal part of the regular but informal meetings, and of what we would call Twelfth-Step calls. Sharing stories reminded the sober members of what it was like and had the best chance of connecting emotionally with the still-suffering alcoholic. The decision to formalize this practice by adding stories to the end of The Big Book reinforced the importance of sharing personal stories as central in A.A. spirituality. Once again we see the experiential nature of Twelve-Step spirituality.

Information about alcoholism does not help a person stop drinking, though it is helpful once one has begun the process of recovery. But stories give hope, communicate love, and build community—which are the power of God, who is love.

Story and Identity

John had been attending A.A. meetings as a result of a court order. He did not appear to be connecting. He was resentful and withdrawn. He never spoke as members shared around the table in the small group. Then after several weeks, one day he began, as is the custom in A.A.

"My name is John; I am an alcoholic. I am glad to be here today."

That was all he said, but it marked a dramatic transition. The other members of the group knew immediately how important this statement was. Until this point, John had continued in denial regarding his disease; now he was beginning to accept reality. He had a disease, alcoholism, that made his life unmanageable. Having recognized this truth, now he was open to learning new ways of living with this disease.

For John this statement was the beginning of developing a new identity. Until this time, John's identity was closely bound to the belief that he was not an alcoholic, that others were overly critical, and that there were many reasons that he "sometimes" drank too much. Now John, in accepting that he was an alcoholic, had to develop a new understanding of who he was, and he would do this by telling his story again and again. Each time he tells his story, new memories of past behavior and new experiences in sobriety will be integrated into his story.

The story usually follows the outline of "what we used to be like, what happened, and what we are like now" (58). As John first began to tell his story, the focus was on remembering past events and incidents that resulted from his drinking. This not only enabled him to remember the pain, shame, and hurt drinking caused, it also allowed him to accept the reality of his disease, often with humor. Laughter is an important part of A.A. storytelling; it defuses the shame of the past and reminds us that the past is past; it cannot be changed.

Much later, on another occasion, I heard John share his story. This time he talked about making amends to his boss at work. As he described it, this was the last thing on earth he wanted to do—to talk with his boss about his drinking. However, his sponsor had been insistent; this was necessary if he were to maintain his sobriety. At the end of the day, he said, this was one of the happiest days of his life. His boss had, of course, known of his poor performance. Now his boss knew why, and there was a new, respectful, and honest relationship between them.

What struck me was the difference between this talk and John's first brief statement. There was an openness that had replaced his fear and protective concealment. There was joy in the new life he was finding. He had developed the ability to accept help; he recognized that this new life was a gift from a power beyond his strength and understanding, which he was comfortable calling God.

In conversation with him after the meeting, he expressed how learning to let go of resentments, self-pity, fear of others, and all those thoughts that go round and round in circles focused on self, has been an added bonus to not drinking. Each day he felt he was growing stronger. He was happier than he had ever been before in his adult life. Finally he was living authentically as the person he truly was and is.

Of course he was involved in the full Twelve-Step program—doing a fearless moral inventory, sharing honestly with God and another human being the exact nature of his wrongs, making amends where possible, working with a sponsor, and attending meetings. But the event that helps John put all this together is when he shares his story. If one were to ask John, "Who are you?" He would reply with his story. "I am an alcoholic who by the grace of God and the Fellowship of Alcoholics Anonymous has found myself in a new life. I am less fearful, more open, more accepting, less needy and dependent, more responsible, more myself, and happy and free." And he would tell his story using concrete examples that "disclose in a general way what we used to be like, what happened, and what we are like now" (58). His account would be filled with humor at the ridiculous actions he often took. He would share painful moments and the time he finally realized he needed help. His story would bring a lump to the listener's throat.

What is true for John is also true for all of us. When asked the question, "Who are you?," we answer best by telling our story.[6] And as we tell our story—seeking to be honest—we gain insight into who we are and what makes us tick.

Our world is in the midst of dramatic change. As we seek to cope with the multitude of cultural, economic, and social changes confronting us today, the issue of selfhood has emerged as a major concern for psychology and sociology. In the 1960s, Erik Erikson developed his theory of psychosocial development and thereby inaugurated concern about human maturation and identity. He is, perhaps, most famous for coining the phrase "identity crisis." Erikson's approach revolutionized psychology. Since the publication of his work, the question of identity has reached a crescendo of urgency.

Who am I?

Psychologist Jerome Bruner draws the distinction between "paradigmatic thought" which seeks to explain through logic, empirical proof, theories, and carefully crafted arguments how the world works, and "narrative."[7] To understand how plants grow or how a computer works, one will need to employ research, observation, and logic. Though I often say my computer hates me because I neglect it and call it bad names, such a story does not actually explain why my computer is refusing to print a particular article. To get my computer to print, I need to get help from someone who understands how computers work. Developing a story of why my computer hates me is absolutely unhelpful.

On the other hand, when we ask the question, "Who am I?," paradigmatic thought is not very helpful. Yes, paradigmatic thought may explain how cells reproduce, how organs work and interact, and how the brain functions, but it does not explain why I do what I do, why I value the things that are important to me, and why I like a particular lifestyle. To answer these questions, we must turn to the narrative mode of thinking.

Why do I care about racial justice? I can only answer that by sharing events and experiences from my youth—a summer on the South Side of Chicago, a summer in the Dominican Republic—my experiences with individuals I have known—a Boy Scout leader, a leader in the church, cohorts and colleagues—as well as my involvement in the civil rights movement.

---

6. A recent summation of the work of many psychologists and sociologists on this topic is found in McAdams, *Art and Science of Personality Development.*

7. Bruner, *Actual Minds, Possible Worlds.*

These stories describe people and events that changed my way of thinking, changed my way of seeing, changed my actions, changed my life. Knowledge about brain function and the endocrine system do not explain my commitment to racial justice.

Narrative mode is used to explain why people do what they do. Of course the narrative must be plausible. It must reflect conceivable human experience. If we are going to believe the explanation of a person's actions, the story must be authentic, it must be congruent with the kinds of thoughts and actions we identify with. If the story seems doubtful and unlikely, it will not touch the emotions; it will not explain the action.

The most important story we ever tell is the story of our lives. Who is the real me? Erikson and others posit that a coherent identity involves having a characteristic pattern of feelings and behavior. "There should be a real you there, an authentic social actor whose dispositional signature is recognizable across a range of social performances."[8] And how does one achieve this recognizable identity? By the construction of a self-defining story: "To be adult means among other things to see one's own life in continuous perspective, both in retrospect and prospect. By accepting some definition as to who he is . . . the adult is able to selectively reconstruct his past in such a way that, step for step, it seems to have planned him, or better, he seems to have planned it."[9]

Identity is, in part, an integrated life story. In psychological science today, investigators use the term "narrative identity" to refer to the internalized and evolving story of the self that a person constructs to provide their life with unity, purpose, and meaning. In formulating a narrative identity, you reconstruct the past and imagine the future in order to explain how you have become the person you are becoming.[10]

We seek a pattern for our lives. So we use a narrative to explain how we came to be and where we may be going. Thus we construct our life story to provide a sense of temporal continuity, to show how our past, as we now selectively recall it, gave birth to the present situation, which will lead to the future as we now imagine it. Of course memory is not an objective tool. Most events in our lives are forgotten. Some events have a dramatic impact on our lives and are embedded in our memories, more or less accurately. Key events in our lives, turning points, insights gained, lessons learned

8. Erikson, as quoted in McAdams, *Art and Science of Personality Development,* 248.

9. Erikson, *Young Man Luther,* 111.

10. McAdams, *Art and Science of Personality Development,* 250.

become central points in our life story. Negative events need to be incorporated into the story with some redemptive meaning. Narrative identity emerges gradually, through daily conversations and social interactions, through introspection, through decisions young people make regarding work and love, and through normative and serendipitous passages in life. As such, our narrative identity provides meaning and verisimilitude more than it provides objective truth.

Over a lifetime our life stories change; our lives change: we marry, we take a new job, we move to a new city or country, we face crises, we overcome hardships, and as we change we revise our life story to include these events. More importantly, our understanding of our lives change, and we need our narrative to include these new understandings. The process of growth is a process of creating a self-identifying life story that in turn creates a new self, all in the context of significant interpersonal relationships and group affiliations. Thus we repeatedly re-create ourselves by telling our story.

The subjective nature of this process is obvious. Memory is selective. Much is forgotten. Current events may trigger memories that had been ignored but now seem important. I believe the health of an individual is directly correlated with openness to incorporating painful as well as enriching events into their life story. Are we open to consider events we would prefer to ignore? Can we find an authentic narrative that includes a truthful acceptance of our life events? One easily recognizes the unhealthy quality of persons who try to maintain an identity that does not reflect their personal history or their basic humanness. They are needy; they are defensive; they are reactive; they are frequently angry; they are often narcissistic; they are difficult to relate to. Developing one's identity by constantly adding to one's life story is a process that continues as long as one is alive. Developing a healthy identity depends on a person's ability to know his or her past as honestly as possible. The truth will indeed make one free.

Alcoholics Anonymous developed its focus on sharing personal stories not because of the research from social scientists but because it worked to assist hopelessly addicted drunks in finding a new identity and a new life. When people repeatedly describe specific events in their lives to others, and when they are reinforced or affirmed for doing so, the stories of these events will be retained and incorporated into a person's developing sense of self.

If we're willing to expose the pages of our lives to the love and understanding of our Higher Power and a fellow alcoholic, we'll surely know a new freedom and a new happiness. We'll discover that love is never having to feel alone again; that God's presence in our lives has become profound; and that the unity of the Fellowship of the spirit can be ours so long as we're willing to 'pass it on.'[11]

Story and Community

One's personal life story provides a sense of identity and purpose. In a similar way, the spirit, the culture of a group may also be described through narrative. For A.A., the language of the heart is central. The alcoholic shares his or her story as honestly and openly as is possible at the given time. The hopeless drunk hears the story, identifies with parts of it, though the details are different. The hopeless drunk finds hope and begins a process of growing through the Fellowship.

The stories have a similarity. They are stories of redemption. Suffering, guilt, despair, anger, and hopelessness have given way to personal enhancement. By the power of God, as God is understood, and the support of the Fellowship of Alcoholics Anonymous, the lost past has been recovered. The storyteller indeed appears "happy, joyous, and free."

In detail, however, the stories are unique. I have a friend who had thirteen DWIs and never went to jail! I suspect that is not a common event in other stories. But as he tells his story, people identify with the crazy danger he and they put themselves and others in. As he tells his story of the surprising intervention of a court that has led to his present sobriety, listeners identify with the miraculous interventions that happened to them. And as he speaks of the new relationship he now shares with his wife, those listening also identify the relationships that have been restored in their lives and which today are healthy and life-giving. Though the specifics are often dramatically different, the stories provide a common identity for the group.

Through the sharing of stories and through listening and identifying with the speaker, the Fellowship comes together and develops its own story. This story gives the community identity and meaning. It is a story of redemption, of hope overcoming despair, of joy overcoming shame, of acceptance overcoming resentment, of power outside oneself overcoming powerlessness, of gratitude overcoming anger. It is a story often told with

11. Chico C., "Building an Arch," 142.

humility and laughter. It is an inclusive story, as the Big Book says, "We are people who normally would not mix" (17). It is the story, not just of a local group, but of the Fellowship. And when an individual hears this story from another individual who is in A.A. and identifies with the teller, this common story provides identity for the individual, for the local group, and for the Fellowship. This common story is powerful and transformative and provides a unity that includes otherness. Again I quote James Nelson:

> The storyteller's autobiographical account provided others with practical advice and encouragement. Perhaps above all it gives a sense of mutual identification and belonging. When in a meeting, my story mentions hidden vodka bottles in my office filing cabinets, heads nod, acknowledging our common insanity. When I tell of my immense gratitude now for a life without hiding, there are smiles of shared thanksgiving. In such ways the little stories of individuals are placed in the framework of the larger story. It is the recovery community's story of what alcoholism looks like and of what makes sobriety possible.[12]

The origin of a group culture or spirit eludes easy, formulaic explanation. It is not likely to evolve from imposed direction, but rather it is a function of the group's shared values, which then filter who will become part of the group. Listening is as important as storytelling in developing the A.A. story. Listening, as discussed earlier, is characteristic of A.A. meetings. Listening involves a kind of surrender. Serious listening involves letting go of the self-assurance that we are right, involves hearing opposing views without seeing them as personal attacks, involves working to understand the other person, and being open to changing not only one's own ideas but also one's values and actions. And when the listener hears his story on another's lips, when the listener identifies with the narrative, then they become part of the group and a new story adds to the shared story.

> One old-timer explained it this way: 'Don't let your mind rattle on at meetings. Then all you'll hear from someone else is something that gets you thinking about what you have to say. Listen to everything the person talking has to say, as if your life depended on it—because it might one day. Listen to everyone this way, especially the ones you want to ignore,' this old-timer said. 'God won't deprive you of the answer you need, if you've come to an A.A. meeting needing an answer. He may, however, have your answer

12. Nelson, *Thirst*, 184.

come out of the mouth of the person you least expect to have your answer.[13]

To be a powerful community requires a shared story. The narrative provides unity and purpose. Community is not so much created as it is discovered.

Because the story is of the language of the heart, words are not always necessary. Words communicate to the mind; the language of the heart, though it uses words, communicates to the spirit. This communication that has power, that touches the emotions, may also come through actions. I know of no better story that illustrates this than the following one from Arizona by a member of A.A. who was taking meetings into the local prison:

> In the beginning the meetings were speaker meetings, but one time the chairperson decided to have a discussion meeting. The chair spoke and then "tagged" the next person to share who then tagged the next and so on. Among the many Native Americans there was one elderly man who spoke no English. A younger Native American volunteered to translate for him,
>
> "I have been here a long time and all because I committed a terrible crime against a brother of mine. I was drunk at the time, but that is not an excuse for what I did because I was drunk a great deal of the time. After I came here [to prison] I started to search for something to relieve the pain I felt for what I had done.
>
> "First I tried the various religions offered here. Then I tried solitary meditations. At no time could I find peace. One evening I heard one of my brethren speak of a meeting that was starting on Wednesday nights. It was a meeting about drinking problems. I came to this meeting. I have been coming back each Wednesday night for over a year. You may ask why I attend a meeting when I could not understand the words that were being spoken. I will tell you.
>
> "From the very first time I stepped into this room and joined this circle of chairs, I felt a powerful spirit. Each time I return here I feel this spirit and the beginning of a wonderful feeling of peace. I need not know the words, although some of them are becoming known to me. All I need to know is that for the hour that I spend here with you people, I am at peace with myself. I feel close to the Great Spirit of my fathers. Words are not necessary. The Great Spirit speaks in all languages. That is all I have to say."[14]

13 "Quiet Guidance."
14. J. F. M., "Circle of Peace," 149–50.

The power of story, the language of the heart, gives all of us our identity. We weave our story from our past, and we use this story to focus what our future will be. The power of story also provides the groups we participate in an identity, a spirit that in turn shapes and molds us, supporting us on our journey. And when the story is truly of the heart, words are not even necessary.

CHAPTER 8

Service

A Twelfth-Step Call

It was during the first months of my recovery in early 1980. Gail and I had just finished dinner when the phone rang. The call was from my sponsor, Jim. All he said was, "We're going on a Twelfth-Step call. I'll pick you up in fifteen minutes." (This was in the days when a sponsor said things like that and sponsees said, "Okay.") It would be my first, but far from my last, such experience.

So, off we went. As we were driving, Jim told me that he had had a call from a woman whose husband he had investigated in his role with the Maryland Department of Motor Vehicles. Jim knew both of them and agreed to have a talk with the man. (Let's call him "Fred.")

I said to Jim, "What do you want me to do?"

Jim replied, "Just do what the Big Book tells us to do—Just tell him exactly what happened to you."

We drove *way* out into the southern Maryland countryside. Eventually we arrived at the house. As we walked up the steps to the front door, I could feel my anxiety rising. Jim knocked on the front screen door. A weak, slurred voice from within said, "Who is it?"

Jim identified himself and said he'd brought a friend with him. "We were in the neighborhood and decided to drop by." (OK, not exactly rigorous honesty—you didn't just drop in where he lived.)

We entered Fred's living room and my anxiety was not lessened by seeing Fred sitting in a recliner with a shotgun across his lap. There was not another stick of furniture to be seen; Fred's wife had left him and taken everything except the chair, the shotgun and . . . Fred.

Jim said, "Fred, what's with the shotgun?"

Fred replied, "I'm protecting my stuff."

Jim looked around the room slowly and said, "Fred, you don't have any stuff."

"Oh, yeah. I forgot," he said and set the gun on the floor.

Jim looked at me with a look that said, "You're on." So, I began to tell Fred exactly what had happened to me. When I finished, Jim did the same. When Jim finished his story, he said to Fred, "Howard and I are going to leave here and go to a meeting of Alcoholics Anonymous. How's about you come with us?"

Fred seemed to think for a bit and then replied, "That's really great what A.A. has done for you guys but I'm not that bad. If I ever do want to go, I'll let you know."

So we thanked Fred for his time and listening. And we left.

As we were backing out Fred's driveway, I asked Jim, "Do you think he'll make it?"

Jim's next words have stuck with me down through the years: "I have no idea. But you and I will stay sober today because we came out here and tried to help this man."

Some 40+ years have passed since that event. I have no idea whatever happened to Fred. Jim, my first sponsor, has long ago gone to the big meeting in the sky. And I'm still sober—still mindful of and grateful for that opportunity of service.

Howard B.

ALTRUISM IS NOT VERY fashionable today. There are voices that would tell us that any act of service is actually done out of self-interest. Helpfulness is often seen as codependence. True altruism, such voices say, would involve a total letting go of self-interest so one's concern is only for the other. This cynical position reinforces a cultural diminishing of the importance of concern for those in need. Since true altruism is impossible, why try to help? Thus volunteer agencies now recruit by telling potential volunteers that helping people will make you feel good, as if the primary motive for doing good is to feel good.

This is a false dichotomy; to assume that self-interest negates the good action of another is to misunderstand the nature of motivation. Motives are always mixed, and self-interest is an important part of any motivation to serve others. If a person seeking to assist another feels no satisfaction or benefit from the action, that person will not be motivated to continue to serve the others' needs. In reaching out to the still-suffering alcoholic, members of A.A. are clear about their motivation: they seek to help the still-suffering alcoholic, *and* they know whatever the active alcoholic does they will still benefit by the reminder of what they were once like. "True morality," writes a member of A.A., "has its inevitable compensations, for when we benefit someone, we increase our own happiness."[1]

This mixed motivation is particularly beneficial when working with alcoholics and other addicts. The drug is powerful, denial is strong, memory is impaired, and blame, rationalization, and resentment together make successful intervention unlikely. The world is full of people—friends, family, co-workers, social workers, preachers—who have tried to help someone who was struggling with alcoholism and given up, resentful of and judgmental about the weakness of the alcoholic. Yet year after year members of A.A. respond to requests to visit someone who is in bondage to the drug; year after year they go with a high degree of success. They persist when others give up because they understand Twelfth-Step calls will help them as well as have the possibility of helping one who is in serious trouble. Lack of success by nonalcoholics leads to burnout. With a member of A.A., the lack of success reminds the person who they were; they know they have gained through the interchange.

Within the culture of Alcoholics Anonymous there is a spirit of service that touches every aspect of the program. The organizational structure is known as "the service structure." People volunteer with a dual motivation: to assist the organization that saved their lives and to help stay sober because service gives meaning to their lives. The board of trustees is titled "The General Service Board," and all those holding office in the service structure are referred to as "trusted servants."

My experience tells me this is not just idealistic talk; service is a central part of recovery. On the many occasions I have called a member of A.A. for assistance with someone who is drinking heavily, I have never been turned down. The responses are very similar: "This is Twelve-Step work, of course I will help." "In A.A. when we are asked to help with another alcoholic, we do not consider if it will be convenient, we act." "I know the answer to your request; it is 'yes.'"

This spirit of service is at the heart of the A.A. Fellowship. They define the program as being built on three legacies: Recovery, Unity, and Service. And they understand that service—whether it is in making coffee or in

1. K. J. C., "Mail Call," 18.

chairing a meeting or in serving as a sponsor or in making a Twelfth-Step call—benefits them as well as others. It provides the opportunity to reinforce the importance of maintaining sobriety and growing spiritually.

I believe if it were possible to act without self-interest, the work would be done poorly and soon not at all. While my primary motive may be to assist the other, if I get nothing in return, after a while I lose all motivation. Loving does not mean one has no needs that desire to be nurtured. Loving means recognizing and accepting one's personal needs and setting them aside in order to respond to the needs of another. Clearly our own needs can get in the way of serving others. I never trust someone who proclaims they are sacrificing themselves as they respond to another's needs. Clearly they have a great need to be admired and honored for their sacrifice. If they are not admired they easily become bitter and burned out, declaring how awful everyone is. True, committed, long-term service will come from one who cares deeply about the person served, but who also profits from the service. At the very least, when we serve others, we find as a by-product meaning and purpose. Bonhoeffer, in a less-well-known passage, denigrated altruism which can become oppressive and exacting. He referred to Christian action as "selfless self-love"[2] which opposed altruism. He did not develop the idea in his writings, but as we can clearly see, even in prison he found a kind of fulfillment. As one who gave his life to oppose Hitler, he understood that selfless giving involved a kind of self-love as well.

This is true in our concern for others; it is also true for our struggles for justice. One of the participants in the Montgomery Bus Boycott in 1955 was a seventy-year-old African American woman known as Sister Pollard. One day, as she was walking, she was asked if she didn't want to ride. When she answered, "No," the person said, "Well, aren't you tired?" She responded, "My feets is tired, but my soul is rested." Sister Pollard understood that her walking for justice healed her soul.[3]

I was fortunate to participate at the conclusion of the march from Selma to Montgomery in 1965. Representative John Lewis described the march in these words:

> The march led that day by Dr. King, was like Gandhi's march to the sea. There was something so peaceful, so holy, so profoundly spiritual about the moving feet on the pavement. As we marched with Dr. King, it seemed like the Heavenly Host was walking with

2. Dahill, "Readings from the Underside of Selfhood," para. 31.
3. King Jr., *Call to Conscience*, 112.

us. We sang. We prayed. One day the rain came down. The skies opened up. The rain could not stop us. We were not afraid. We truly were, as the Negro spiritual goes, "wadin' in the water." We were God's children, wadin' in the water." [4]

I sought to express similar thoughts in a letter to my parents. "I would characterize the march as a combination of a football game, a Santa Claus parade, and a Baptist revival. There was a feeling that simply because they were allowed to march and because the march was so strongly supported that victory had already been won." One important aspect of Dr. King's leadership was his understanding that the experience of standing together for justice must also be an experience that heals the soul. Self-interest does not negate service; self-interest often supports service.

As with all of the insights of Twelve-Step spirituality, this approach was learned through experience. After Bill W. had his white light experience in the Towns Hospital, he began to carry the message of his and Ebby's recovery to other alcoholics, but none sobered up. As he described these efforts:

> "My spiritual experience had been so sudden, brilliant, and powerful that I had begun to be sure I was destined to fix just about all the drunks in the world . . . I kept harping on my mystical awakening, and the customers were uniformly repelled."
>
> His chastening came from the beloved Dr. Silkworth,
>
> "Quit preaching, quit harping on your odd spiritual experience. Tell your own story. Then pour it into those drunks how medically hopeless alcoholism is. Soften them up enough first. *Then* maybe they will buy what you really have to say."[5]

Bill speaks of the arrogance and imprudence of this approach, which in effect said, "You must be as I am, believe as I believe, do as I do." Preaching, advising, or judging simply do not work to intervene with an alcoholic's behavior. Bill goes on to say he followed Dr. Silkworth's advice at his meeting with Dr. Bob in Akron. Thus was the Twelfth-Step call discovered, and Alcoholics Anonymous born.

Central in the Twelfth-Step call is the sharing of one's personal story: one drunk sharing with another his own story as honestly and as completely

---

4. King Jr., *Call to Conscience*, 113.

5. The story of Bill's immediate actions following his spiritual experience is told in many different places. This version is found in Bill W., *Language of the Heart*, 247 (italics original).

as possible, treating the other with respect and understanding. Howard's story illustrates the guiding principle: one makes the call and then lets go. We cannot control or force others to accept help. Over the years it became clear that even if the call does not change the behavior of the drunk, in making the call the sober alcoholic reinforces his or her own resolve to stay sober.

The importance of honestly sharing one's own story and then respecting the choice of the individual can hardly be overstated. If advice or urging or preaching helped, A.A. would never have been needed and would not exist today. Betsy S., in sharing her story, describes this clearly in relating what happened to her:

> Finally, when I was approached by those who lived in sobriety, I sensed they had a real solution. They weren't "better" than me. Indeed they were just like me. And I sensed that if I could just put my false pride away, they could actually begin to teach me how to live. How to stop, not only drinking, but my crazy way of thinking. Always trying to plot and plan my next move. Always having a "better" idea. That was so incredibly difficult. I began to really surrender to an idea. I realized that it was because of *me* that my life was ugly.[6]

Loving without a Price Tag

This does not mean that outcomes are unimportant. Clearly whether or not Fred gets into treatment and attends A.A. makes a great deal of difference to him—preventing insanity, incarceration, and/or death—and to those around him who end up dealing with the consequences of his disease. It makes a difference if Fred drives while intoxicated. It makes a difference what he does with his shotgun. Outcomes are important.

The problem comes when we are too committed to the outcome and begin to try to compel others to follow our agenda. Focusing on results invites the ego to take over. When desire to help becomes desire to be successful, we will seek to control, manipulate, and force the other to do what we believe is best for him or her. The idea of respecting the other person and letting go so they can make a decision disappears. The focus on success interferes with the possibility of reaching the goal. Nowhere is this more evident than with the members of the alcoholic's family.

6. Betsy S., "In Shambles," 39.

Addiction is a family disease in that members of the family are affected spiritually and emotionally. A spouse or significant other may spend their energies trying to get an active alcoholic to stop drinking or trying to control their actions. Children growing up in an alcoholic family may have spent much of their lives struggling with unfair criticism, chaotic behavior, constantly shifting standards, and the necessity of keeping all this secret. To be emotionally involved with an active alcoholic or addict is to experience deep and long-lasting hopelessness and despair.

Al-Anon developed because friends and family members of the alcoholic, like the alcoholic, need help dealing with this cunning, baffling, and powerful disease. In the early days of Alcoholics Anonymous, spouses of alcoholics often found themselves together in the kitchen of a school or church while waiting for their alcoholic partners to end their meetings. As they talked, they discovered a commonality in how they had been affected by living with an alcoholic. They too needed help and turned to the Twelve Steps of A.A. as a model for recovery. Soon family groups began to develop around the nation. In 1951, the name Al-Anon Family Groups was selected. The Twelve Steps and Twelve Traditions were soon adapted and adopted.

The Al-Anon Steps also begin with Step 1: that we are powerless and our lives have become unmanageable. I quote from my friend Caroline who is a longtime member of Al-Anon and describes with rigorous honesty how one's life goes out of control:

> My side of the disease isn't about the obsession over the next drink, or the next hit. My side is all about obsessing over the drinker, the addict—Is he drinking?, Is he upset?, Will he be able to keep his job?, Did he have a drink before driving the kids to baseball practice? What if? What if? What if? Before Al-Anon I kept my eyes and heart on the addict at all times like a bulldog refusing to release. Even when I didn't want to think about him, I was unable not to think about him. My sense of safety and well being were completely wrapped up and dependent upon how he was doing.

This focus on the alcoholic/addict has additional consequences for one's behavior. Alcoholism is a disease of relationships as well as a physical addiction. Driven by the need for the drug, the alcoholic rationalizes, blames, deceives, breaks promises, hides, and uses many other creative ways to diffuse responsibility for their actions and maintain the supply of alcohol. The people who are involved with the alcoholic react to their behavior. They try to control it, make up for it, and/or hide it. They often blame themselves for it and are hurt by it. Eventually they become emotionally disabled themselves. Again, my friend Caroline describes this experience of how the obsession with the drinker affected her life:

> So many of us feel guilty or even shameful if we aren't 'helping.' If we aren't in the middle of someone else's affairs, we may feel we aren't worthy of love and belonging. . . . we have to face how we have hustled to feel worthy of other people's love. Will they love me if I'm not 'helping' and telling them what to do? [Doesn't] loving someone and caring about them [mean] looking after them and keeping them safe when they've proven they can't make good decisions?

Step One, when truly accepted, which is as difficult for the family members as it is for the alcoholic, begins the process of healing. "Letting go of the illusion of control over other people, their actions and their addiction to alcohol, we find an enormous burden is lifted, and we begin to discover the freedom and the power we do possess—the power to define and live our own lives."[7] Coming to recognize what and who we are responsible for and what and who we are not responsible for is freeing and empowering. This insight is often summarized in Al-Anon by "the three Cs: I didn't cause it; I can't control it; I can't cure it."[8] Recognizing that one cannot force a person not to drink, we come to understand that trying to force, manipulate, or otherwise control another person violates the integrity of the person. Though the intention may be to protect the individual, controlling behavior mostly produces a negative reaction. Two principles develop: the only person one can hope to improve is oneself, and don't do for others what they can do for themselves.

These two principles are important for all our relationships. While in the addicted family seeking to control and manipulate becomes extreme, they may also damage relationships in all sorts of situations, as is illustrated by this story from Haim Ginott's *Between Parent & Teenager*:

> While strolling on the beach, Nora, age twenty-one, asked her mother, "Mom, how do you hold a husband after you finally get him?" Her mother thought for a moment, bent down and took two handfuls of sand. One hand she squeezed hard; the sand escaped through her fingers. The tighter she squeezed, the more sand fell to the ground. The other hand she kept open; the sand remained.

7. *Paths to Recovery*, 9–10.
8. *Paths to Recovery*, 8.

Nora watched her mother; she said quietly, "I see."

Nora had been quarreling with her fiancé and was feeling miserable. Her mother's silent message gave her insight. To herself, she thought, "I am too possessive. I force issues. I need to change."

Later that week Nora and her fiancé were driving to dinner. He was angry. She recognized his anger and realized she had accepted the invitation and had pushed him to come with her even though she knew he disliked this couple. It occurred to her that she had often forced him into things he did not enjoy.

She put her arm around his arm, "I want to apologize. I understand how you feel. You just don't care to be around this couple. I'm sorry I pushed you to come."

He looked at her in surprise. His anger dissolved. "Well, . . . thanks for being understanding." The evening was not great, but it was a lot better without his anger, for everyone. [9]

This still leaves the problem of outcomes. It matters a lot whether or not the alcoholic gets help and finds sobriety and recovery. We know advice, judgment, seeking to control, talking down to, manipulating, or otherwise attempting to change the alcoholic's drinking and behavior results in negative, defensive reactions by the alcoholic and personal damage to the one seeking to help. On the other hand, we know that doing nothing accomplishes nothing, and the disease continues to progress. The Twelfth-Step call process of not judging but sharing and then allowing the active alcoholic to make a choice, while not always successful, frequently is. The same goes for the Al-Anon approach of letting go: while it does not always lead to the alcoholic's seeking help, over time it frequently does. Clearly, when confronted with addiction, we must act, but to do so is extremely difficult and a positive outcome is not automatic. How can we "let go and let God"? How do we keep emotional attachment at bay? How can we reign in our ego and act with compassion?

My first response to this concern of how to let go and let God is the fact that we never know the actual outcome of any of our attempts to help. An intervention may seem unsuccessful, but only the future will show us what happened, and even then we may not see the result. The following story from Ron N. of Oakhurst, California clearly shows one never knows what may come from an attempt to help:

> I was standing outside before the Sunday night meeting when a car pulled up and a woman got out. She was nicely dressed, appeared

9. Ginott, *Between Parent & Teenager*, 215–16.

to be in her mid thirties. She went over to the passenger's side and opened the door, reached inside, grabbed a wet drunk, and pulled him out. He could hardly walk. All she said was, "I don't want him anymore. You take him."

I got a friend from the meeting to help me. The man was really bombed, slurring his words, reeking of booze, and was dirty and unkempt. We took him to my friend's home. He seemed to want to go to a hospital and be admitted to its alcoholic ward. We both thought he had done this many times before.

So off we went on the one-hour drive to the hospital. He kept wanting to kiss us. His breath was terrible. We got to the hospital; there were many people in the waiting room. Finally the doctor began to interview him, and we went outside for some fresh night air. It was almost midnight. Twenty minutes later we went back in to find out if he would be admitted. We could not find our drunk. Another patient said he had taken off through the exit door real fast. He was gone, gone, gone. We stopped for breakfast and got home about 3:00 AM.

We never heard from this drunk, nor did we see him at any meetings. I ran into the woman who had dropped him off. She told me he had moved to the East Coast and was really drinking there.

About five years passed. One day I got a message on my answering machine thanking me for my help that night. This fellow had been sober in A.A. for two years. I got the message on Christmas Day—what a present![10]

Sometimes interventions can be successful immediately; sometimes it appears that we have been totally irrelevant. I've learned from my friends in A.A. that in any effort to help you do the best you can and then leave the results in the hands of God and the other. It is never a waste of time and effort. While we do not know what to expect when we seek to intervene, we do know what will happen if the person continues to drink alcoholically: they will be arrested or lose the ability to function and be committed to a mental hospital or die. Or as A.A. members often say, "They will be locked up, screwed up, or covered up."

There is, however, a larger question concerning how, in the face of challenging tasks the individual stays motivated to act. It would be so much easier to ignore the problems. To begin to examine this question, let's look at Step Twelve. "Having had a spiritual awakening as a result of these steps,

10. Ron N., "You Take Him," 74–75.

we tried to carry this message to alcoholics, and to practice these principles in all our affairs."

First, I believe the fundamental character of the spiritual awakening one has as a result of the steps is the movement from being self-directed—I can control my drinking, I am strong, I will control you—to being directed by a power greater than self. It is a movement toward recognition that we are not God, we cannot control our life or the lives of others, and that seeking such control actually makes life unmanageable. It is a movement toward letting go of all that baggage and accepting that we must find a new way of living that is directed by a Higher Power. The spiritual awakening is about living life on life's terms, living in the world as it is and not trying to make the world conform to our needs and expectations.

Second, this spiritual awakening does not come primarily through personal reflection and study; it comes through interaction with a group of persons struggling with the same issues and concerns. What enables a person to reach out to the still-suffering alcoholic by making a Twelve-Step call is a group where there is a spirit of honesty and truth, where members share their personal stories, and where powerlessness is recognized, owned, and accepted.

I believe effective involvement in service depends on such a spiritual awakening. The service may be a ministry to other individuals, or it may be an effort to address injustice in our society. Whatever the service one pursues, the effectiveness will largely depend on the spiritual strength of those involved. If we take the model of Twelve-Step spirituality, we will look for a community that will support the project, and we will expect to learn and grow spiritually from our involvement. When in Step Eleven we ask for knowledge of God's will for us and the power to carry that out, the act of asking makes us aware of our powerlessness. We are not in control. We need help. We cannot fix the problem. But we can make a difference, usually as part of a larger community. To act in service requires a healthy self-love and a large dose of humility.

While I was Rector of Trinity Church, Buffalo, the congregation founded Homespace, a transitional living facility for homeless single-parent families. Inaugurated in 1987 by the vestry, through a series of meetings with the parish, we determined housing was the area where we were called to act. A group of about twenty formed a committee, and after two years of study and meetings, they recognized the need for housing for homeless single parents and their children. Along with the housing, a program was needed to provide assistance in learning the skills for independent living. We joined with the historically African American St. Phillip's Church as the plans began to emerge. Some cultural differences nearly broke this coalition apart. Finally, in the early nineties, funding for the facility and for the program developed with the aid of state and federal resources. In 1994, Homespace opened. Later, another facility called Second Chance was developed. Seven years it took; seven years is a long time to keep a group motivated. I believe we were successful in large part as a result of another member of the church staff, the Rev. Ellen Montgomery, who met with the group each month, leading theological reflection to keep us on track, seeking first God's will and God's power to carry it out. The group and the regular spiritual reflection provided the necessary support and motivation.

In a world where outcomes matter, in a world where the forces that diminish human lives are immense, complex, and powerful, how do we act and yet keep our ego and desire for success from sabotaging our efforts? First, we recognize that we cannot control outcomes. Then we recognize we need help. Third, we find or develop a group to assist us with these insights. And then, finally, we are empowered to act, together.

Accepting Limitations

At the heart of Twelve-Step spirituality is the acceptance of human limitations. It begins with the first step: "We were powerless over alcohol," and we were unable to manage our own lives. We needed help. The first step is to accept our weakness, and it is in this acceptance that we will find our strength. I believe this may be the true genius of this spiritual program. Acceptance of weakness and limitations opens the possibility of a new life based on honesty, self-revelation, group support, service, humility, and the possibility of wholeness.[11]

The Third Tradition, "The only requirement for membership is a desire to stop drinking," reflects this acceptance of limitation. One joins A.A. because they desire to stop drinking, but they are unable to do so alone; help is needed.

This acceptance includes the limitation that the alcoholic cannot promise to never drink alcohol again. This promise to abstain is unrealistic. It is too difficult, and it represents the many broken promises the alcoholic has made over the years. But he or she can refrain from drinking today.

11. This theme is a primary premise in Kurtz, *Not-God*.

"One day at a time" represents acceptance that the alcoholic cannot stop the preoccupation with alcohol and the loss of control after the first drink, but for twenty-four hours he or she can restrain from taking that first drink.

This theme of acceptance of human limitations undergirds other aspects of this way of life. Members accept that perfection is not only an unachievable goal, but as a goal, perfection causes much personal difficulty and interpersonal conflict. Though A.A. began as part of the Oxford Group meetings, they soon found the Oxford Group culture was uninterested in drunks and the "four absolutes"—absolute honesty, absolute purity, absolute unselfishness, and absolute love—were damaging to their spiritual journey. Focusing on perfection meant focusing on self, and the "bondage of self" is a major part of the spiritual problem. Thus the phrase found in chapter 5 of the Big Book, "How It Works," has become central in understanding the Steps: "The principles we have set down are guides to progress. We claim spiritual progress rather than spiritual perfection" (60).

Recognizing that, to find sobriety and health, the alcoholic must have help from a power outside the person, A.A. is clear that this power may be called "God," but seeking to define God brought conflict and dissension. Thus "Higher Power" and "God of our understanding" define that power which is beyond human definition.

Anonymity is likewise an important part of accepting limitations. Those who do not understand A.A. often think anonymity is about hiding in shame because one is weak and unable to control drinking. Perhaps in the beginning that may have been true, but it is clear that "anonymity is the spiritual foundation of all [A.A.] traditions" (Tradition Twelve). Grandiosity is a common aspect of the active alcoholic's personality, as it is with many of us who are not alcoholic. We who are grandiose have dreams of great success. At the heart of those dreams are our supposed skills, talents, and contacts—our self-inflated importance and opinion. Grandiosity is a common symptom of self-will run rampant, and when the alcoholic sets himself or herself up as the savior, it is not uncommon that he or she decides they are strong enough to take a drink now and then. The result is disastrous. Anonymity underscores the principle that, as limited human beings, members are not world-renowned reformers.

> It is essential for my personal survival and that of the Fellowship
> that I not use A.A. to put myself in the limelight. Anonymity is
> a way for me to work on my humility. Since pride is one of my

most dangerous shortcomings, practicing humility is one of the best ways to overcome it.[12]

The importance of human limitation is also seen in the structure of Alcoholics Anonymous. Just as the individual is made whole by accepting his limitation, so too the organization of A.A. is careful to incorporate many practices that are based on the recognition of the dangers of authority becoming absolute or arrogant. In the beginning there were discussions of owning hospitals and treatment centers as well as licensing addiction counselors. The membership strongly opposed such actions. What had saved their lives was one drunk talking to another. This understanding that led members to accept their limitations then informed the importance of human limitation for the A.A. Service Structure. The groups are autonomous (Tradition Four). The organization is to be nonprofessional (Tradition Eight). Involvement in issues other than sharing the news of recovery with other alcoholics is to be avoided (Tradition Ten). Self-support (Tradition Seven) prevents bending principles to raise money. Even as a Trustee (nonalcoholic), A.A. will not accept my financial contribution, as I am not a member. To prevent anyone from accumulating too much authority, all positions have term limits, and one cannot be reelected when the term is completed. The structure provides a model for "servant leadership." Authority is in the annual conference composed of delegates from every area in Canada and the United States. The goal is to achieve substantial unanimity on all actions, and the minority voice is always heard, even after a motion has passed. Just as acceptance of human limitation is the beginning point for recovery of the alcoholic, so acceptance that A.A. cannot solve all human problems, but is limited to the nonprofessional sharing, informs the structure.

Given this focus on human limitation, one can easily see why Twelfth-Step calls are carried out as they are. The recovering alcoholic knows they are unable to fix every active alcoholic. The recovering alcoholic also knows the sharing of his or her story about the obsession and destruction of alcohol provides a nonjudgmental invitation for the active drinker to seek this new way. By accepting their weakness, they have something to give, and they can give it without excessive expectation or ego involvement. The spiritual transformation founded on acceptance of human limitation enables the person to give without any price tag attached.

12. *Daily Reflections*, 340.

> Through experience with Twelfth Step work, I came to understand the rewards of giving that demands nothing in return. At first I expected recovery in others, but I soon learned that this did not happen. Once I acquired the humility to accept the fact that every Twelfth Step call was not going to result in a success, then I was open to receive the rewards of selfless giving.[13]

Humility is not a word one often hears at A.A. gatherings. But humility is essentially what we are discussing. Humility begins with the acceptance of one's being human, not God, or in Dr. Tiebout's words, "giving up reliance on one's own omnipotence."[14] Humility is based on honesty. It does not exaggerate or minimize. It accepts life as it is and the self as we are. It is the opposite of self-exultation and the opposite of self-abasement. Humility does not make comparisons, does not ask whether I am first or last. Coming from a spiritual awakening, this ability to accept our limitations, to accept the world as it is, and to accept ourselves and others as we are, provides the basis for the saying often seen or heard in Twelve-Step groups, "love and tolerance is our code." Humility is the deep acceptance that our fundamental value is that we are human beings, and the recognition that our power comes from outside ourselves—from others and from God.

> By being humble I realize I am not the center of the universe. When I was drinking, I was consumed by pride and self-centeredness. I felt the entire world revolved around me, that I was master of my destiny. Humility enables me to depend more on God to help me overcome obstacles, to help me with my own imperfections, so that I may grow spiritually.[15]

Humility brings a kind of simplicity. Humility simply accepts being human, accepts our world as it is, and learns how to live with self and others and how to enjoy this life. Comparisons are unimportant; *what is* is what's important. Humility allows us to see so we can put first things first. Above all, humility accepts and understands how much we receive from others. Humility is the foundation for love and tolerance.

13. *Daily Reflections*, 363.
14. Tiebout, as quoted in Bill W., *Language of the Heart*, 99.
15. *Daily Reflections*, 202.

Why Service?

Human beings may be the only animal that, recognizing we will die, seeks to find some meaning in life. We seem to be particularly equipped to explore the question, "Does my existence have any purpose?" We make choices and reflect on whether or not they are the best choice for us. We delay immediate gratification for greater good. We take advice from friends and people we consider authorities. We spend a lot of energy on feelings like guilt, joy, resentment—seeking to sort out how to improve our character. We have the ability to learn from our past and to learn from others. We find meaning in our employment, in caring for our family, in being involved in civic life, in our churches, or in the many other activities that fill our lives. We also find ourselves distracted from these activities that provide meaning by other activities—television, social media, sports, finances, and the like—that are enjoyable and entertaining and may serve to help us relax or that may be just filling up time.

> If all life consists of is working all day, then sitting in a bar for hours, or coming home to sit in front of the television until overtaken by sleep, then [our] capacity for abstract thinking, meditation, and philosophizing is a complete waste.[16]

For the alcoholic in A.A., service brings meaning to one's life. The Twelfth-Step call is an important part of meaningful service, but so is serving to help set up a meeting, greeting newcomers, being involved in the service structure, taking meetings to prisons or rehab hospitals, or in many, many other ways seeking to extend the hand of A.A. to the still-suffering alcoholic. Having discovered the joy of life free from the bondage of addiction, free from the bondage of self, free from the isolation, loneliness, and guilt, in gratitude they wish to make that freedom available to others. As the Big Book says:

> Life will take on new meaning. To watch people recover, to see them help others, to watch loneliness vanish, to see a fellowship grow up about you, to have a host of friends—this is an experience you must not miss. . . . Frequent contact with newcomers and with each other is the bright spot of our lives. (89)

What is true for the recovering addict is true for all of us: service in the broadest sense is how we find purpose in our lives. Serving others, seeking

16. Twerski, *I'd Like to Call for Help,* 39.

to change unjust social structures, is not easy. Easy is getting discouraged, burning out, giving up. Serving requires time and commitment. Distractions easily erode our commitment. Twelve-Step spirituality provides some clues that can assist us as we push through discouragement to engage with perseverance.

First, we accept our limitations; acceptance of human limitation is critical to service. Ironically, such acceptance empowers us even in the face of overwhelming odds. When we let go of our need to be successful, when we act because there is a need, even though we feel inadequate, we will make a difference. As we realize our success is less important than our acting, we experience the moment when we serve without success as a primary goal, when we love without a price tag.

> Several years ago a teacher who taught children in a large city hospital received a call requesting that she visit a particular child. She took the boy's name and was told by the teacher on the phone, "We are studying nouns and adverbs in his class now. I'd be grateful if you could help him with his homework, so he doesn't fall behind the others."
>
> It wasn't until the visiting teacher was outside the boy's room that she realized it was located in the hospital's burn unit. She entered the room and found a young boy horribly burned and in great pain. She felt that she couldn't just turn around and walk out, so she awkwardly stammered, "I'm the hospital teacher, and your teacher sent me to help you with nouns and adverbs."
>
> The boy was in such pain he barely responded. She stumbled through his lesson, ashamed at putting him through such a senseless exercise.
>
> The next morning a nurse on the burn unit asked her, "What did you do to that boy?" Before she could finish her apology, the nurse interrupted her: "You don't understand. We've been very worried about him. But ever since you were here yesterday, his whole attitude has changed. He's fighting back, responding to treatment—it's as though he's decided to live."
>
> The boy later explained that he had completely given up hope until he saw that teacher. It all changed when he came to a simple realization. He expressed it this way: "They wouldn't send a teacher to work on nouns and adverbs with a dying boy, would they?"

It is the irony of grace: in so far as we are able to act, let go of the ego, and trust that every action makes a difference, we will make a difference and will personally know peace and joy. Ego-driven actions that are successful invite us to take the credit, puff ourselves up, and assume we are in control. Such ego-driven activities are heading for a fall. Humility invites us to keep it simple: there is a need, we have some ability and experience to respond to it. We do not have the ability to make particular outcomes happen; we cannot solve the problem; but by the grace of God and the support of other concerned persons and the support of the community to which we belong, we can make a difference. Instead of an inflated ego, we end up with a sense of purpose and excitement over small incidents of progress.

Second, we must continue to grow spiritually. At a minimum, God's will for us is to let go of the self-focused need to control, to live in the world as it is and not as we might seek to create it in our minds, and to serve others because we recognize their worth as human beings, having discovered our worth as a human being. As we grow in this spiritual journey from self-direction to being open to live in the world as it is, our eyes are opened and we see the beauty of creation, the beauty and needs of those to whom we are connected, and the possibilities for service. We move from self-focus to a healthy self-love and acceptance. As I learn to love myself in a healthy and honest way, then I am able to love others, as they are, and to serve them in healthy, not needy, ways. This is what is meant by "let go and let God."

> As long as I am acting in a loving and caring manner, I am not responsible for how others react. This frees me from pleasing people at my own emotional expense.[17]

Such self-reflection takes us to Step Eleven. We seek to nurture our conscious contact with the God of our understanding, seeking only knowledge of the divine will and strength to carry it out. Service comes through the spiritual transformation that begins with openness—accepting limits and letting go of control. Now we can begin to accept ourselves as we are and see others as they truly are as well. As we humbly recognize our own shortcomings and character disorders, we accept that we are of worth, not because we are God's gift to the world, but because we are human beings, beloved of God. As we humbly accept ourselves, honestly and with humor, we will also accept other imperfect, limited, anxious human beings. Love and tolerance become more than just our code; love and tolerance become the way we view ourselves and others.

Finally, we need help. Just as no one can discern truth individually (chapter 5), so too no one can truly accept himself or herself in isolation.

17. R. M., "An Equal-Opportunity Deplorer," 23.

No one can recognize the mixed nature of their own personal motivation. Since none of us is omnicompetent and omniscient (i.e., God), we need others for insight, knowledge, support, and motivation. Help is readily available in a multitude of groups. For those caught by the disease of alcoholism, there are A.A. and Al-Anon. For others there are a variety of groups one can join, or one can develop a personal support group. The spiritual life is a journey we take with others. It is a journey in which we fall down, are helped up, and then someone else falls down and we help them up.

Humor is a great tool for bursting one's grandiosity and inflated ego. Every A.A. meeting I have attended has been filled with laughter. Stories of grandiose schemes, stories of self-inflicted disasters, stories of lucky breaks—all allowing one to laugh at human fallibility. The combination of our inflated egos and actual events is often ridiculously funny, but what is humor if it is not shared?

When we accept the reality of limited control, when we accept our imperfections, when we accept that we do not have control over our lives, that is the beginning of our ability to truly serve others. Such acceptance is the foundation of a powerful spirituality. Now we can see that we share with all people the reality of anxiety, limitation, and imperfection. Now we can begin to accept ourselves as we are and see others as they truly are as well. As we humbly accept ourselves honestly and with humor, we will also accept other imperfect, limited, anxious human beings. We are free—free from the need to be perfect, free to accept and work with others, free to serve even when success seems impossible, free to work to bring others to this new life of service and joy, and free truly to love.

CHAPTER 9

From Hope to Gratitude

TWELVE-STEP SPIRITUALITY BEGINS WHEN one is caught by the hope that life can be better, that one can be free from their present prisons and find meaning through service to others. From hope one moves to gratitude, but it is not immediate; it usually takes years. The transformation passes through times of discouragement, through learning to deal with fear, through learning to ask for help, and finally to a sense of the giftedness of life.

Hope

Working with alcoholics and addicts, working in areas of social justice, involvement in issues around climate change, seeking to support persons who are struggling to find spiritual and emotional health—all of this easily leads to discouragement. The problems are large; resistance and inertia are strong; desired successes may seem few and far between. One can easily become pessimistic and cynical. Pessimism and cynicism nurture discouragement; they do not assist one in their efforts.

As part of our motivation we must distinguish between optimism and hope. When Howard and his sponsor, Jim, made their Twelfth-Step call, they were hopeful that it would make a difference to Fred, that Fred would accept that life had become unmanageable and that he needed help. That does not mean they were optimistic this would happen. But if there were no hope, then they would not take the time. Without hope why would anyone spend valuable time seeking to intervene? Hope and optimism are distinctly different realities. Optimism believes with or without evidence that things will get better. If they do not improve, the optimist feels defeated.

Hope depends on past experience. Jim and Howard knew that alcoholics can respond to another alcoholic and seek help, discover support, and begin recovery. The basis of their hope is their memory. That Fred seems uninterested does not change that foundation for hope. They have seen people change in the past. They remember that they themselves, in response to an intervention, changed and found a new life. Because others took the time to intervene in their lives, they know it can be effective. Their own story provides a solid foundation for hope.

Toward the end of his life, Martin Luther King Jr. said that he was not optimistic, but he still had hope. He had seen how nonviolent resistance had brought dramatic change, but he also saw how deeply established structural racism was, and is, in our society. We can understand his discouragement. His hope, however, was based on strong realities. He knew they could effect change because they had done so. King's hope was based on his experience that, standing together, they could open the eyes of others who were offended by discrimination and injustice. His hope was also based on his absolute faith in God's support and call. He frequently expressed this faith in God's providence with these words, "the arc of the moral universe is long, but it bends toward justice."[1] His call was to continue until a new social structure emerged.

> The only normalcy that we will settle for is the normalcy that recognizes the dignity and worth of all of God's children. The only normalcy that we will settle for is the normalcy that allows judgment to run down like waters, and righteousness like a mighty stream. [see Amos 5:24] The only normalcy that we will settle for is the normalcy of brotherhood, the normalcy of true peace, the normalcy of justice.[2]

Hope, not optimism, motivated his words and action.

This distinction between optimism and hope is essential for any who seek to work in service to others or work to see the vision of a just society begin to come into existence. While I am generally optimistic and while I believe progress for individuals and for society happens, at times I feel like the world is coming apart, and there is no progress for those who suffer. At such times I find I must search for a strong basis for hope.

---

1. From Dr. King's speech at the conclusion of the Selma to Montgomery march, March 25, 1965. See King Jr., *Call to Conscience*, 131.

2. From Dr. King's speech at the conclusion of the Selma to Montgomery march, March 25, 1965. See King Jr., *Call to Conscience*, 129–30.

Working with alcoholics and working to understand apocalyptic literature in Scripture has provided me with a foundation for hope that combines experience with faith.

For families where there is substance abuse, holidays are particularly stressful times. Dad fell asleep at the table, again. Aunt May got in arguments, again, with every member of the family. Jim had an automobile accident, but the police officer let him off with a warning; the car can be repaired. Grampa was drunk and knocked over the Christmas tree. At the country club Mary spilled her drink down the front of Ethel's new dress and then vomited all over the carpet in the reception area. In every case the perpetrator had excuses and the witnesses decided to let it go—holidays should be happy family times.

In A.A. and N.A. it is common to remember and celebrate the date when a member had his or her last drink or drug. January and February have an abundance of these anniversary celebrations, often referred to as "birthdays." In the open meeting I sometimes attend, we have around a dozen regular attendees. In February, three of them celebrated their anniversaries; two others celebrated in January. We had lots of wonderful cake in that group this winter.

Holiday disasters and A.A. birthdays have a direct and obvious connection. Addiction is a progressive disease. The progression is not a straight line, but involves many behavioral ups and downs as the person loses control and the drinking takes over. The holidays provide a number of opportunities for inappropriate behavior, and families and colleagues often come to the end of their endurance. Enough is enough! It's never been this bad before. It's time to get help!

In the beginning of the alcoholic's progress into addiction, the family lectures seem to help; the policeman's warning seems appropriate; the supervisor's confrontation seems to have positive results. But as the addiction worsens, those affected become less and less able to control the drinker, and the drinker finds it is more and more difficult to control his or her drinking. Finally things get so bad, change must happen. We can only hope that change involves intervention and treatment for the addict and for the significant others.

While it is counterintuitive, hope comes for the addicted only as things get worse. For the family of an alcoholic, one of the most hopeful aspects of the holidays may well be the disasters that occur because of the addict's drinking or drugging. Life simply must get worse before a person is willing to give up and ask for help. As strange as it may sound, things getting worse precedes and prepares a basis for hope.

As I studied apocalyptic literature, I discovered that this understanding for when we can be hopeful is also the basic understanding of hope in apocalyptic literature.[3] In Daniel, beginning with the seventh chapter, we have the accounts of the progression of oppressors, each worse than the previous, until the end when "there shall be a time of trouble, such as never has been since there was a nation till that time; but at that time your people shall be delivered" (Dan 12:1). In Revelation, five times John tells the story of redemption describing it in seven incidents. In the first six incidents the world goes from bad to worse until the seventh incident describes divine intervention and victory. The apocalyptic literature was popular among people who suffered and for whom there appeared to be no hope. Their understanding of hope was that "getting worse" is a sign of a new world coming.

We find the same phenomenon in the civil rights movement. In April 1963, King and the Southern Christian Leadership Conference began a campaign in Birmingham largely because segregation there was among the worst in the nation. There, Eugene (Bull) Connor, using dogs and a water cannon against the demonstrators, provided visual images on television that shocked the world. The result was integration of the downtown merchants and soon, under strong pressure from local organizations, all public facilities including the schools. This horrific confrontation raised King to the status of a national leader and empowered both local and national movements for integration.

As I am writing, demonstrations are occurring throughout our country and in many other parts of the world, protesting police violence against African American men and women following the death of George Floyd at the hands of a Minneapolis policeman. George Zimmerman was acquitted in 2013 in the shooting death of Trayvon Martin in Florida. Though the Black Lives Matter organization predates the event, since that time they have become more visible nationally in raising the issue of police violence against Black Americans. As the number of deaths at the hands of police has received publicity, the number of demonstrations has increased largely as a result of their work. The numbers are staggering; the incidents, startling. Public support for the organization and message of Black Lives Matter has

---

3. Ewing, *Power of the Lamb.*

moved from under 40 percent to over 65 percent.[4] Systematic racism and violence against Black Americans has been ongoing since the days of slavery. Why has the level of concern suddenly increased so dramatically? Why now? There are many answers to this question, including the prevalence of phone videos that provide incontestable evidence. However, at least part of the reason is the clarity that George Floyd's death has laid bare. Despite the progress from the civil rights movement, despite the increase in political power minorities have gained through voting; despite electing a Black president, the systemic racism, the violence, the deaths continue. Liberty and justice were supposed to be becoming more equitable. It's time to change.

Sometimes things have to get worse before they can become better. As we watch things become less and less healthy—individuals, organizations, government, social norms—we can have hope. When it gets bad enough, they will have to change.

Another basis for hope, as discussed in chapter 6, can be found in the power of a healthy community to transform social structures. A healthy community can also transform individual lives. Addiction is a lonely disease. As the disease progresses, the addict/alcoholic separates from many friends who would seek to help by controlling his drinking, and friends who once hung out with the alcoholic begin to separate from him or her. Behavior produces chaos, and the alcoholic/addict becomes defensive, lies in order to defuse criticism, and allows anger to grow. Isolated with a life that has become unmanageable, it is no wonder that depression dominates. As the disease progresses, most contemplate and many attempt suicide, perhaps the most desperate act of hopelessness. Much of the spiritual crisis for alcoholics can be found in this aloneness.

Where is the hope? Certainly not in the ability of the alcoholic to change behavior and overcome depression. The hope is found when the alcoholic connects with another human being.

> Our success with each new prospect has always rested squarely on our ability to identify with him or her in experience, in language and especially in feeling—that profound feeling for each other that goes deeper than words. This is what we really mean when we say "one alcoholic talking to another."[5]

---

4. Pew Research Center, "Amid Protests."
5. Bill W., *Language of the Heart*, 293.

The importance of honestly sharing one's story is the possibility that the alcoholic, in hearing the other's story, identifies with the pain, the chaos, the sense of powerlessness, and the despair. Connecting depends on identifying, not on changing, attitudes or behavior, or even stopping drinking and drugging. Some who begin attending A.A. continue to drink for some time, continue nursing resentment and anger, and continue trying to control others and manipulate difficult situations. Change is not instant; current brain research tells us it takes approximately two years for the brain to reprogram and heal the damage caused by addiction.[6] But the nonjudgmental connection of one person to the other begins a process that can lead to a new life.

The connection begins the process of overcoming the isolation of the disease. The connection involves the first surrender—the recognition that as limited human beings we cannot fix ourselves; we need others. Thus my friend Jean's statement that what kept her coming back to meetings was that someone told her at her first meeting, "You will never be alone again." Connecting is where the process begins. The memory of being isolated and then connecting with another human being provides the hope needed for a person to continue to go to meetings, get a sponsor, work the Steps, and reach out to help others.

I view recovery as a process by which a person who has been isolated reconnects to human society, usually through a small group. I have hope whenever a person who is part of a healthy community connects with someone who is isolated and in trouble. Change takes time, actually a lifetime, but the process begins when the two people connect. This connection occurs most profoundly in the context of vulnerability: when people can share honestly, despite fear or shame. This explains why Twelve-Step spirituality has proved to be successful with so many addictions—cocaine, narcotics, overeating, gambling, etc. One person honestly and vulnerably sharing their story connects with another who identifies and begins a process of recovery, a process of reentering human society through a group composed of other people who have experienced the same bondage but yet now are happy, joyous, and free.

6. Hazelden Betty Ford Butler Center for Research, https://www.hazeldenbettyford.org/education/bcr.

Fear

Fear is a primary destroyer of hope and action. Fear, like so many human emotions, plays a helpful role but may also play a destructive role. Fear is helpful when it makes us aware of danger and results in recognition of actions we can take to avoid the danger. But fear can also paralyze a person so that they cannot take appropriate actions. Fear can so preoccupy a person's life (e.g., a parent) to the point where it damages important relationships (e.g., parent and child). Fear can transfer from one thing to another (e.g., loss of job to fear of migrants). Fear can infect a group and turn a valid concern into a despised menace. Fear moves us to focus on self, and not in a healthy way, but rather in an anxiety-driven way.

As I am writing, our world is struggling with the COVID-19 pandemic. At this time the primary response we have made is to encourage (or seek to enforce) social distancing and quarantine. We gather as groups through electronic means. I meet each Sunday with a group from the church I attend. Each Sunday, no matter the given topic, the discussion moves to sharing the sense of isolation and loneliness we are feeling being unable to gather as a community. The A.A. group I am connected with stays in touch via phone and texting. Again there is a deep sense of isolation and loneliness we are feeling being unable to gather as a community. Electronic media provides some connection, but loneliness and isolation are being felt by many, particularly those who live alone.

While fear of contracting COVID-19—personally or by someone we love—is upon us now, there are constant fears that are with us always: fear for ourselves, fear for those we love, fear for our social structures, fear for our world. Fear is the basic recognition that we cannot depend on the world to be a safe place. The issue is not "Can we rid ourselves of fear?"; the issue is "How do we live in a world with so many fearful things? How can we live with fear in a way that is spiritually healthy?" We use a lot of unhealthy approaches: denial, anger, blame, and paralyzed inaction. Does Twelve-Step spirituality show us how to live with fear in healthier ways?

One of the ways we deal with the current fear—in fact one way we can always deal with fear—is to connect with others. Since fear drives us to focus on self, one way to tame fear is to connect with others, reducing the focus on self and opening one up to alternative perspectives and ideas. Seeking to deal with fear without help is a way of encouraging the emotion to grow stronger. Sharing our fears with another who is an understanding listener provides a way to live with fear. As we live through this pandemic, we recognize there is a true danger in contracting the coronavirus. But the fear has produced some strange behaviors, from depression to violation of appropriate standards of social distancing. These behaviors emerge, at least in part, because we have been forced to distance ourselves from others who are part of important communities in our lives.

While social media may not be as effective as face-to-face gatherings, clearly it can lead to being connected and to strengthening relationships. The history of letter-writing gives us another confirmation that we can connect in ways other than face-to-face meetings. We are limited human beings who need each other, and in times of isolation we need to find ways to connect.

My friend Jan, who lives in Canada, sent this email to several of us:

> I just wanted to share some news that really brought a smile to my face. Each Monday night at 8 PM my home group, the Forest Lakeside Group, meets for a closed discussion meeting. We have been meeting by zoom during this COVID crisis as well. We have had a young man, James, with us for several weeks now and he shared with us this past Monday night that he is 32 days sober. He has been attending zoom meetings and staying sober. Well if that's not a miracle in itself I don't know what is. It brought tears to my eyes. He can't wait to meet us all in person. And the feeling is mutual.

Being a part of something, having a community and connectedness, is an antidote to fear.

When I work to encourage people to get involved in programs that seek to support others who are in need or that work to build a more just and equal society, the most common response I receive involves a lack of time. For many that is legitimate; for others it is an excuse, hiding the fear that we will not be successful, that we will waste our time and produce limited results. Dare we seek to respond to the challenge of finding housing for the homeless? Dare we seek to work in the area of addiction and alcoholism— the number one health problem in the United States? Dare we try to assist a family where there is spousal abuse? Dare we work to end gun violence in our country? The problems we confront are so vast and so complicated that even small progress seems unlikely. Fear of failure is an important reason people do not get involved in service and working for change. Why try if we know we will fail?

Fear of failure is present with all of us because we have all failed at one task or another. While I am not a student of self-help literature, I have read some and have not found any references to dealing with fear of failure. The solution to failure in our culture seems to be to let it go, to rationalize, and to try harder. How many times have we heard the story of Thomas Edison, who tried a thousand possibilities before he made a successful incandescent light bulb? Most of us carry the memories of our failures in that part of the brain where we store secrets not to be shared. They are unnecessary burdens that prevent us from taking creative and important action.

If there is any group on our planet that knows how to deal with failure, it is the members of Alcoholics Anonymous. Beginning with the failure to control their drinking, they often move on to failed marriages, failed business careers, and failed friendships. Their way of dealing with failure is helpful to any of us willing to follow it.

Dealing with failure begins with rigorous, honest acceptance of what happened. As I learned from friends in A.A: one thing we have to accept is that we cannot change the past. As long as our failures are secrets, they will not go away. As I accept the past, I begin to acknowledge my feelings of failure, of anger, of sorrow, and of victimization. And as I express those feelings, slowly the truth of what actually happened begins to emerge. My memory of the failure when all the feelings were attached is often dramatically different from my memory after I have processed the feelings. Then I am able to begin to see my role in what happened, the role of social structures or patterns, and the role of others involved. And when I discover I am carrying resentments against the others who were involved, I try to follow the advice I have learned from A.A.—to pray for the people that have caused the resentment (sage advice sometimes delivered with simplicity: "Pray for the sons of bitches."). It is a simple task, and it produces surprising results.

In A.A., this is all worked out with the help of a sponsor, with the help of others sharing their stories with honesty and humor, and through the personal sharing of one's own story. In the words of Lisa N.,

> The Fifth Step was the closest I'd ever gotten to being that real to another person. More than just a confession of my faults, it was also a way of showing someone my feelings and fears. . . . The program tells me that in order to recover I must be willing to develop a manner of living that demands rigorous honesty. So when I retire at night, I ask myself: Is there something that I should discuss with another person at once? What do I not want to share? Do I feel any guilt? Am I worried about something? Fearful? What was my thought-life like today? These questions spur me to talk

to someone. The more I share, the more I live in integrity; and the more I live in integrity, the more at peace I am with myself, and the more useful I can be to God and my fellows.[7]

Imagine someone who, despite the obvious impossibilities for success, operates with no apparent fear of failure or of those who would oppose her. Greta Thunberg, the eighteen-year-old Swedish activist calling upon governments throughout the world, seems to have little fear of failure. At fifteen, concerned about climate change and the nonaction by government, she began skipping school on Fridays to demonstrate at the Swedish Parliament. Her parents were supportive. I suspect she simply felt the need to act, ignoring the question of whether or not she might make a difference. Then others joined her, and now, as we know, this has expanded into a worldwide movement involving students all over the globe. She was *Time Magazine's* Person of the Year in 2019. She has addressed heads of state at the UN, met with the pope, sparred with the President of the United States, and inspired 4 million people to join the global climate strike on September 20, 2019, in what was the largest climate demonstration in human history. Clearly she did not know this would happen. She saw a critical problem, and although she was only one, young, small person, she decided she had to do something. Most of us would never begin such a crusade for the fear we would fail. What can one powerless person do? We are yet to see what change will come from her effort, which is being overshadowed by the COVID-19 pandemic. I believe she has made, and will continue to make, a difference—all because one young girl acted with integrity despite obstacles.

One may think of Rosa Parks as another example. True, she had participated in training for nonviolent resistance at the Highlander Folk School, but when she refused to give up her seat on the bus, it had more to do with being tired of abuse than with a plan to begin the civil rights movement. Facing one's fear and still acting with integrity can be a major force for change. It is not our omnipotence or competence that makes change happen. God gives us a vision of a better way. God gives us discomfort at our failure as a people to live the better way. We are called to act and leave the results in God's hands.

To be an activist one must face fear and, with whatever help they can find, act with integrity. We never know what the future may bring. Dr. King understood that dealing with fear was a test of faith. "Our capacity to deal creatively with shattered dreams is ultimately determined by our faith in

7. Lisa N., "As Real as I Can Be," 56.

God. . . . However dismal and catastrophic may be the present circumstances, we know we are not alone."[8]

Resentment

> Resentment is the "number one" offender. It destroys more alcoholics than anything else. From it stem all forms of spiritual disease, for we have been not only mentally and physically ill, we have been spiritually sick. When the spiritual malady is overcome, we straighten out mentally and physically. (64)

This statement out of *Alcoholics Anonymous* seems astounding to those of us who are not recovering addicts. Perhaps we should pay attention. The understanding underlying recovery in Twelve-Step spirituality is that to maintain continued abstinence from the crutch that cripples, one must grow to become more spiritually healthy. Like the Holocaust survivor who still resents the Nazis, one who is filled with resentment is still in prison.

Resentment etiologically means "to feel again." This is why resentment is so damaging to spiritual growth—it keeps a person focused on the past and on their perception of being victimized. For example, an employee gets a somewhat negative annual performance evaluation from his supervisor. Immediately he assumes she is overly critical, is prejudiced toward men, and is trying to show her supervisor that she can be a strong manager. Resentment is born with the denial that this is about him, but rather it is about her. Denial, however, does not change the facts about his performance and the possibility that this is a first warning. So he is stuck. To reduce his resentment he first needs to understand his role in why he received a negative evaluation. What has he done or not done and what can he do differently? Not wanting to accept responsibility for his own actions, however, he revisits the evaluation, telling himself how unfair it is, blaming his supervisor, and slowly building a case that he is being victimized. Over and over he stews in his resentment. She is unreasonable; he is one of the best employees the company has; he should be in charge, not her; she should be home taking care of children. As a victim, there is nothing he can do to free himself—it's all her fault. He goes over and over the injury; revisiting the hurt, the powerlessness, the fear, the feeling of being wronged. He is stuck.

---

8. King Jr., "Shattered Dreams," 256.

His focus is on the past and upon himself. One can easily see how for a sober alcoholic this whirlwind could lead to a drink.

For any of us who seek to grow spiritually, this concern about resentment is helpful advice. Resentment isolates us, focuses us solely on our hurts, our desires, and our victimhood. We are imprisoned in our own painful past.

How are we to deal with this spiritual malady? First, we take our inventory: what was my role in what happened? The other may be at fault, but how did I participate in the events? As we begin to get a more objective picture, we must share our perception—with a sponsor, a friend, someone who is outside the situation and therefore neutral. Bringing our own part into the light transforms the situation. Spiritual growth comes when we work to rectify our defects of character, not when we focus on the past faults and failings of others. We get unstuck when we focus on the future and on self-improvement, when we accept the event as it actually happened and forgive ourselves for our part in what happened, and when we accept the other person with as little judgment as possible.

We are on a journey from our initial hope that life can be better to gratitude for all the gifts we have received. Resentment is, indeed, a huge pothole in the road.

Listening

In the popular mind, A.A. meetings involve someone sharing his or her story. While in speaker meetings this is true, equally important is the fact that everyone else is listening. In discussion meetings the norm is for a person to share briefly without interruption and then another will speak. We do a lot of listening in A.A. There is no cross-talk, no debating, just brief sharing and intense listening. The goal for those listening is to find some aspect in the sharing with which they can identify. This process is not written down in some sort of rule book; it is simply how it works. Listening is how we connect. For the speakers, respectful listening helps them to open up and speak more freely and honestly. For the listeners, letting go of personal concerns is how belonging is cemented.

Listening is powerful because it involves a kind of surrender. It involves letting go of one's personal agenda and seeking to understand the person who is speaking. It means accepting and, when possible, identifying with the other's feelings—anger, joy, sadness, fear, excitement, and shame.

To listen carefully, one must enter into the other's experience of weakness and powerlessness, must share the other's vulnerability. I find listening to be much more work than sharing. And on top of all this, listening often does not feel like it is useful.

There are many ways in our everyday lives we avoid this style of listening. We immediately think of personal experience and take control of the conversation with a me-too-ism—"I used to do the same thing." We argue or disagree with the speaker. We give advice: "You just need to work harder." We try to fix the problem: "I know a good doctor who is good with your concern." We become moralizing and judgmental, in tone if not in words. We become uncomfortable when heavy emotions are expressed in tears or in anger, so we cut off the conversation with cheap consolation: "I'm sure everything will turn out just fine."

Letting go of personal comfort and personal opinions in order to listen carefully is, frankly, difficult. Truly it is a gift to listen to another; it is one of the most demanding gifts we can give someone. At times one may feel that listening may not be effective; the listener seems passive. However, because it is truly a gift, it is very powerful. It is a most effective way we connect to each other.

> Early in his sobriety Ralph was struggling. He was resentful, frustrated, and upset. As he was about to go out to his old haunts, he remembered the saying, "Call before you fall." So "I picked up the phone and called an A.A. friend, who suggested I come to his house and talk about it.
>
> "He listened to me all night as we sat and drank coffee, although he seemed unable to come up with a solution. I began to notice light coming through his windows. It was Sunday morning, and suddenly I no longer felt a desire to party or be resentful of my wife. I thanked my friend and returned home, sober. . . .
>
> "It took me quite a few years to realize the spiritual experience I had had—God had restored me to sanity and kept me sober for another day.
>
> "That was forty-five years ago."[9]

Listening is one of the most powerful gifts we all have to give to others.

9. Ralph B., "Call Before You Fall," 51–52.

Gratitude

One result of accepting that we are limited human beings is to gain the humility to recognize that who we are comes from people and forces outside ourselves. One result of acknowledging and accepting our limits is that this act of humility opens one up to connect with others, whether it be family, other people with similar challenges, or perhaps an experience of God for those that have such faith. One result of accepting personal limitation is to recognize the large number of people who have played significant roles in forming the person we have become.

Twelve-Step spirituality is helpful to all of us because all of us suffer from addictive behavior. Such behavior is very different from the physical/mental addiction to alcohol or drugs. However, the tools of Twelve-Step spirituality are just as helpful in healing addictive behavior as they are for healing physical addiction.

I am a workaholic. I have been accused by some of my closest friends of seeking to be omnicompetent. In my ministry, I accepted positions where institutional survival was questionable and the challenge to continue was large. In addition, I'm a wood worker; I build furniture. I do construction and remodeling of our 180-year-old house, including electrical, plumbing, carpentry, and tile work. I keep my to-do list on the computer. And I seem never to have enough time. Retirement has been a good thing for me. It is forcing me again to take inventory, to come to understand my character defects, and humbly to ask God to remove them. I hope that I am a recovering workaholic.

Why do I seem so addicted to accomplishment? I find it difficult to understand, but I know that in my past I substituted admiration for friendship. Today I know that I am loved—by my wife, by God, by my brothers, by a few close friends. Still, somewhere deep within this wounded soul there is a person who feels his worth depends on his accomplishments. I am a beloved child of God; I am a loving husband and father; that should be enough. And at times it is. At those times I know the freedom of self-acceptance; then I can share my vulnerability; then I know my limitations.

But at other times I focus on my past failures. I feel like I should have done something else. I once again struggle with a sense of failure and shame. I'm back in that self-focused belief that I should fix myself as well as fix everything else. So for me one aspect of God's will is the letting go of my need to be omnicompetent and in charge. Sometimes this is as simple as asking for help. Sometimes it is as challenging as letting go of the fear of failure. Sometimes it is the need to let go of the desire for answers where there are no answers. When we are able to let go, ask for help, accept our fears, live with ambiguity, we open ourselves to the love that surrounds us, and we live in this world as it is, which includes our limitations.

As we grow in this spiritual journey from self-direction to being open to live in the world as it is, our eyes are opened and we see the beauty of creation, the beauty and needs of those to whom we are connected, and the possibilities for service. We move from self-focus to a healthy self-love and acceptance. As I learn to love myself in a healthy and honest way, then I am able to love others, as they are, and to serve them in healthy, not needy, ways.

At a minimum then, God's will for us is to let go of the self-focused need to control, to live in the world as it is and not as we might seek to envision it; and to serve others because we recognize their worth as human beings, having discovered our worth as a human being. Letting go of the self-focus is the way we become free.

I have come to understand that all of life is essentially a gift, not what I have accomplished. What have I actually received that is not a gift—my intelligence? The love of my wife? My home? The love of my children? The opportunity to serve, be it in the church or the Fellowship of Alcoholics Anonymous? Even my sense of motivation? All of these were gifts from my parents, the church that raised, loved, and challenged me, and the mystery that allows anyone to love me—all gifts.

As long as I am under the bondage of self, as long as I think I can accomplish anything I desire, as long as I seek to be omnicompetent, I will not, I cannot, receive these gifts with gratitude. When my hands are so tightly clenched because of my earnest desire to accomplish, then it is impossible to receive anything. Life is a gift; that's the meaning of grace—it is unearned, undeserved, freely given. Such is life. And as I let go of the self-focus, I become able to see the love that surrounds me on every side. When I no longer believe (unconsciously) that I must accomplish, when I recognize my limitations and know that I cannot do all things, then I will have time. Insofar as we are able to surrender, to let go of our self-focus, we will be free from the bondage of self and will live in gratitude for all the gifts we have been given which we now thankfully receive. A dominant part of my experience with members of Alcoholics Anonymous is their sense of gratitude, even gratitude for the illness of alcoholism which brought them into the spiritual program of Alcoholics Anonymous.

Of course it does no good to tell someone to let go. We can try as hard as we are able to let go of our self-focus, but the very act of trying is itself focused on self. It has been said that the true sign of humility is that the person is unaware of being humble. Letting go, surrender, turning our wills and our lives over to the care of God as described in Step Three, is not something we can achieve by our efforts alone. When that happens, that too is a gift.

Perhaps this explains why so many alcoholics describe their recovery, as well as that of others, as a miracle. Recovery is a miracle because it did not result from personal effort; it happened as the result of a variety of coincidences or events that shaped time. All the active alcoholic had to do was surrender all that self-focused effort, accept that they could not control their life, go to meetings, get a sponsor, and work the Steps. When one considers how life was before and how it is now, what happened to bring the change feels and looks like a miracle:

> I got sober by the grace of God on January 1, 2000 after three years inside the system where I'm serving double life. I was only 17 years old when I was arrested for my crime, which was the result of my alcoholism. As a result of other A.A.s in prison, I was given a firm handshake of what A.A. really is and how to find the way to a better life. I've found purpose, usefulness, and meaning in the Fellowship. I've had some wonderful sponsors and sponsored some wonderful men. I'm simply a drunk to whom God has given some great gifts. I show my gratitude by sharing them. I share me by my defects! The age of miracles is still here. If a juvenile with double life can get Twelfth Stepped by other convicts and have as beautiful a life as I have in spite of my situation, anything is possible! No one is too hopeless for the power of our message.[10]

We live in a world that is filled with fear and grace. Our world is not a safe place; it is filled with complex, powerful, and entrenched institutions and cultures, some of which are destructive to creative human life. But those in recovery understand that our world is also filled with persons who are happy, joyous, and free—persons who extend hands to us by sharing in our vulnerable and fearful lives. Love surrounds us on every side. We do not earn love; we do not achieve it by our actions. Only by accepting our limitations do we become connected with others. We are not God, and we need others who also understand they are not God. Recovery is a process

10. William W., *Sharing from Behind the Walls*, 2.

of spiritual growth that begins when we surrender and accept help from powers outside ourselves.

Gratitude comes because we (humbly) recognize how much of who we are has come from the efforts and gifts of others. By the simple repetitious practice of reviewing one's gifts daily, gratitude evolves into a working part of the individual's perspective. Gratitude acts as a preventative against taking credit for who we have become. To have a grateful heart is to be focused on the gifts we have received, to be free from the bondage of self. Humility and gratitude may be primary characteristics of recovery; they are also the characteristics that allow us to love sincerely and honestly. Following a presentation Bill W. felt later was driven by the desire for applause and approval, he wrote:

> How much better it would have been had I felt *gratitude* rather than self-satisfaction—*gratitude* that I had once suffered the pains of alcoholism, *gratitude* that a miracle of recovery had been worked upon me from above, *gratitude* for the privilege of serving my fellow alcoholics, and *gratitude* for those fraternal ties which bound me ever closer to them in a comradeship such as few societies of men have ever known.[11]

Gratitude orients us outside ourselves and toward others. It is more than a feeling; it is a spiritual quality that affects all of a person's life, as this story illustrates:

> "Rebbe, we are puzzled. It says in the Talmud that we must thank God as much for the bad days, as for the good. How can that be? What would our gratitude mean, if we gave it equally for the good and the bad?"
>
> The Maggid replied, "Go to Anapol. Reb Zusya will have an answer for you."
>
> Arriving in Anapol, [the Hasidim] inquired for Reb Zusya. At last they came to the poorest street of the city. There, crowed between two small houses, they found a tiny shack, sagging with age. When they entered, they saw Reb Zusya sitting at a bare table, reading a volume by the light of the only small window. "Welcome, strangers!" he said. "Please pardon me for not getting up, I have hurt my leg. Would you like food? I have some bread. And there is water!"
>
> "No. We have come only to ask you a question. The Maggid of Mezeritch told us you might help us understand: Why do our

11. Bill W., *Language of the Heart*, 36 (italics original).

sages tell us to thank God as much for the bad days as for the good?"

Reb Zusya laughed, "Me? I have no idea why the Maggid sent you to me." He shook his head in puzzlement. "You see, I have never had a bad day. Every day God has given to me has been filled with miracles."[12]

Gratitude frees us from self-focus, resentment, anger, and despair. Gratitude enables us to accept ourselves as we truly are, to accept others as they truly are, and to accept the world as it truly is. Gratitude allows us to forgive and love—ourselves and others. Gratitude allows us to experience awe.

"Wow" and "Thanks!" are always in some sense prayers of gratitude. When I see the cedar waxwing birds devour the fruit of our serviceberry tree in a single day, I wonder: How did they know to come on that day? How did they know there were berries on the tree? When I see the flowers on my rhododendron plants open, I wonder: Do they really need to be so full and so beautiful to attract the bees? Would not a simple single flower be sufficient? When I take my wife's hand as we walk through the woods, I wonder: Why does it matter so much and feel so right to touch? How did we ever come to love and care for each other?

"Wow" and "Thanks!" involve being free from self-focus; we look at a marvel and exclaim "Wow!" When another listens to our joy or our pain, our "Thanks" takes us away from self to appreciation that another cares. Awe and gratitude come as we recognize there is some force or reality greater than the abilities of self that surrounds us on every side if we have the eyes to see. Humility and gratitude are both the fruits and states of recovery. Wow!

---

12. Kurtz and Ketcham, *Experiencing Spirituality*, 270–71.

CHAPTER 10

To My Friends in A.A.

Thank You

During my drinking years, my one and only concern was to have my fellow man think highly of me. My ambition in everything I did was to have the power to be at the top. My inner self kept telling me something else but I couldn't accept it. I didn't even allow myself to realize that I wore a mask continually. Finally, when the mask came off and I cried out to the only God I could conceive, the Fellowship of A.A., my group and the Twelve Steps were there. I learned how to change resentments into acceptance, fear into hope and anger into love. I have learned also, through loving without undue expectations, through sharing my concerns and caring for my fellow man, that each day can be joyous and fruitful. I begin and end my day with thanks to God, who has so generously shed His grace on me.[1]

THE DAY I FIRST read this passage from A.A.'s *Daily Reflections*, I was stunned. If one removed the reference to alcohol, this was my story. I was caught in the bondage of substituting admiration for love. I immediately read it to my wife, who agreed that this is a brief telling of my story. It was the church that, by loving me (not knowing my need for achievements), made it possible for me to accept that love is a gift I could never earn. I was loved as I am, and all I must do is accept that to find a new life of grace. My story is a story of freedom moving from a bondage I helped create to an

---

1. *Daily Reflections*, 350.

acceptance that I needed help. No wonder I identified with so many members of Alcoholics Anonymous. No wonder the spiritual program of the Twelve Steps has provided me with a guide to greater and greater health. Church members generally do not want their leaders to be rigorously honest. Clergy groups too often are superficial, focusing on ecclesiastical issues rather than personal concerns. I was truly blessed by that small group of alcoholics that I met with every Tuesday afternoon for five years. I found a group that only wanted rigorous honesty. I have had a variety of sponsors over the years. While I am not a member of A.A., I have been welcomed and supported by this culture of honesty, spiritual growth, and gratitude. I do not believe my bondage to achievement is the same as the physical bondage of addiction, but the spiritual program of the Twelve Steps has proved to be as transformative for me as it is to all who go to meetings, get a sponsor, and work the Steps.

So to my friends in A.A., I say thank you. A.A. has one purpose: to carry the message of hope to the alcoholic who still suffers. It does not exist to assist clergy in dealing with their stress. Thank you for allowing me to be part of this amazing organization. Thank you for allowing me to serve the Fellowship. Practicing the Twelve Steps and being present to the Fellowship has nurtured my spiritual growth, has strengthened my relationship with the God whose name and nature is love, and has provided spiritual support for me, personally and professionally. I have learned to be free—free especially from the fear of being honest. And with that freedom has come happiness. I continue to let go of those things I cannot change, especially the self-pity and feelings that are attached to dwelling on the past. I continue to grow with concern for others being more central. Humbly, I say thank you.

Challenges

For obvious reasons my descriptions of the A.A. Fellowship may, at times, seem idealistic and uncritical. The gifts of Alcoholics Anonymous, the transformative power of its principles and process, are remarkable. Working these principles and process has seeded new life for millions of alcoholics and their families. Similarly, other fellowships that have sprung forth using the same twelve steps, principles, and process have given new life to individuals in them. This does not, however, mean that the organization does not face certain issues and challenges. Times have changed since 1935, when Bill W. used the technology of his day—the telephone—to make the call that led him to Dr. Bob. Today's technology is dramatically different. Further, the organization has grown from a few small groups into a worldwide movement with millions of active members. With growth and changing times come new challenges and the need to respond appropriately. As a nonmember who is a friend of A.A., with over forty-five years involvement in the Fellowship, I feel compelled to examine some of the challenges presented by these changes and suggest how we might respond to the new scene, keeping the mission central. I believe today's responses are embedded in the culture and history of the Fellowship. What follows is a brief review of some of the challenges being faced today, concluded by my thoughts on how we can respond.

The Twelve Steps were designed to outline a program of action through which the alcoholic can find personal sobriety and freedom. The Twelve Traditions are principles that outline how groups relate to each other and to the whole. They were borne from the early mistakes of AA's founders and early members. The unity that results from groups working within the guideposts of the Traditions is vital to Alcoholics Anonymous. The long form of the First Tradition states clearly why unity is so important: "Each member of Alcoholics Anonymous is but a small part of a great whole. *A.A. must continue to live or most of us will surely die.* Hence our common welfare comes first. But individual welfare follows close after" (emphasis added). In the A.A. literature, unity is one of the three legacies that is vital to the health, existence, and purpose of the Fellowship. Should A.A. be divided by controversy, the power and strength of the program would be deeply compromised.

"God" Talk

As an ordained clergyman who has spent his life in the church, direct talk of "God" is not unusual, uncomfortable, or foreign to me. That said, I recognize the freedom of belief in A.A. to be broad, inclusive, and incredibly tolerant. Possibly because of my background, and I hope because of my tolerant nature, the concern I have been most involved with in A.A. has been the use of the term "God" in the A.A. literature and at A.A. meetings. As described earlier, from the beginning there has been concern about the use of God in the program. Thus the terms "Higher Power" and "God as we understood Him" were used to describe the power that allows the alcoholic to be released from the bondage of addiction. The literature is very clear that the definition of God can be as broad as a person desires. As I perceive how God operates in A.A., we are talking about experience, not theology. Thus one might speak of the God of our experience instead of the God of our understanding.

A.A. is a spiritual program; it is not religious. But there is a danger to this tolerance if religion sneaks in. It is common in many parts of the country to end the meeting with the Lord's Prayer. The use of the Serenity Prayer is also common. When a meeting includes prayers and a lot of God-talk, we run the risk of excluding some who come seeking help and are turned off by religious language. We often hear stories of people who were turned off by the God-talk when they attended their first A.A. meeting. They returned because they had no place else to go. Many later found a God of their understanding that supported their new life. We do not, however, hear the stories of those who were turned off by the God-talk at their first meeting and who never returned to A.A. One can only fear they never found help.

Membership in A.A. is defined by the Third Tradition, "The only requirement for A.A. membership is the desire to stop drinking." We have a single primary purpose articulated in the Fifth Tradition, "to carry [the] message to the alcoholic who still suffers." Part of what has always been an attraction of A.A. for me has been it's openness to anyone who desires to stop drinking. Before other organizations were open to Black Americans, other minorities, women, or gay & lesbian persons, A.A. welcomed them. This record of inclusion is dramatic, and comes from the Third Tradition. I do not understand how anyone might be excluded because of theology. This Fellowship has always found unity through love and tolerance, not through theological agreement.

In November of 2014, I was privileged to be a speaker at the First International Conference for Atheists, Agnostics, and Free Thinkers in A.A. Many seemed surprised that I, as a religious, nonalcoholic person whose spiritual life has been strengthened, sustained, and enriched by this Fellowship, would be part of this group. Frankly, I was surprised by the exclusion from A.A. felt by many of the participants in the conference. I was unaware of the depth of pain experienced by so many who were told they could never stay sober unless they came to believe in a God of their understanding. Clearly that conclusion is not true, as I have met many with thirty, forty years sobriety who do not believe in "an anthropomorphic, interventionist (male) deity." As one participant expressed his experience, "You would be surprised by the scrutiny (be it reality or perception) that nonbelievers are subject to within A.A. at large. Some of our fellow A.A. members are fearful, dismissive, or outright hostile towards us." The frequent advice is to fake it until it becomes real; what a dramatic violation of the standard of rigorous honesty this is!

The spirituality of the Twelve Steps, and of A.A. as a whole, is clear and powerful. Hope, truth, honesty, letting go, acceptance, loving others as a way of loving self, gratitude—these are spiritual realities that are part of the culture of A.A. One might also mention unity, carrying the message, singleness of purpose, self-support, and anonymity as spiritual characteristics. These qualities form an invisible, intangible culture; they are spiritual realities. They are difficult, maybe even impossible to define; we must experience them. This invisible culture, this spirit of A.A., is what changes and forms the lives of the members. This is experiential spirituality. It is pragmatic. It is known through living, not from some preordained theoretical position. What truly matters is this spirituality: a newcomer caught by hope, the sharing of one's story seeking above all to be truthful, letting go of the desire to be self-directed by choosing a sponsor, identifying with another who is both different and yet the same, discovering the gifts we have been given, becoming happy, joyous, and free—all made possible by the spirit of A.A.—unseen, indescribable, known through experience.

I find that believers, nonbelievers, theists, atheists, agnostics, and free-thinkers all share common ground found in a common experience that is shaped and formed by this culture of A.A. This collective power of A.A. is greater than any particular person or group; it makes the impossible possible. This power can be discovered within a person, but it is also beyond. It is an inner resource; it is a collective power.

Many in A.A. refer to this invisible reality, this culture, this spirit, this higher power, as God. Others who cannot bring themselves to compromise their rational understandings to believe in some sort of deity still experience the power of this invisible reality within A.A. groups. I would suggest that since all the members of the Fellowship are influenced by this invisible power, the differences between those who wish to call it God and those who choose a different name are tiny in comparison to the shared experience. What we believe about something is far less important to living than what we experience. Experience is what transforms us; belief is our attempt to explain the experience. Experience trumps explanation. I believe the dialogue between those who are religious and those who are free-thinkers, agnostics, and atheists in A.A., can bear much fruit. And I believe the common ground of experience provides the basis for that conversation.

By now it is clear that I believe maintaining the separation between religion and the spirituality of Alcoholics Anonymous is critical to the primary purpose of carrying the message of hope to the still-suffering alcoholic and for the unity of the Fellowship. Some newcomers need God-based recovery, while others need secular recovery; can traditional A.A.s and secular A.A.s work together to create groups and a fellowship that works for both?

I do believe as long as the separation between religion and spirituality is maintained, those who are comfortable in church, synagogue, or mosque will find that resources within the religious community can strengthen their spiritual journey. Singing, for example, opens the heart and soul in ways no other activity can. That's why singing was such an important part of the civil rights movement. To join in a familiar hymn or a moving anthem helps one experience that they are not alone, that they are surrounded by a loving power. We don't sing in A.A., and that is as it should be. But I would be spiritually less whole if I did not go to church regularly for the singing. Spiritual direction is another tool religious communities may have that is available to those who desire it. Prayer and meditation are not easy; a spiritual director is like a specialized sponsor and can be very helpful as we seek to improve our conscious contact with God. In fact weekly attendance at a religious community may be an important part of improving our conscious contact with God. For some A.A. members, attendance at meetings achieves the desired fellowship and connection needed in order to be spiritually whole.

I hope the reader is hearing my deep desire that the members of the A.A. Fellowship—both those who accept belief in a traditional God and those who identify themselves as atheists, agnostics, and free-thinkers—relax. All share a common experience of powerlessness and empowerment. All share the common purpose of carrying the message. And all care deeply about the unity of this life-giving organization.

In the words of a friend who identifies himself as an atheist:

> the God concept creeps into the picture when Wilson states what the Big Book is all about: "Its main object is to enable you to find a power greater than yourself which will solve your problem." (Big Book, p. 45). He concedes the search for this power may be difficult but, "Much to our relief we discovered we did not need to

consider another's conception of God." (Big Book, p. 46). I knew I was not willing to accept any conception of God! Would that disqualify me from membership? Wilson says no. "You can if you wish make itself your higher power." (12 and 12, p. 27). Whether he intended to or not, Wilson had conflated the term higher power with the word God and accorded me the option to designate the fellowship as my higher power. I call it the agnostic loophole, and now I had a humanist foundation upon which to build my recovery—one day at a time. Wilson went on to say he knew of many alcoholics who began their recovery journey using the fellowship as their higher power . . . "And most of them began to talk of God." (12 and 12, p. 28) What was noteworthy to me is that he did not say "all of them."[2]

Finances

On February 8, 1940, after a month of preparation, John D. Rockefeller Jr. sponsored a dinner at the Union Club, having invited 400 of New York's wealthiest to learn about this new approach to dealing with alcoholism. Less than five years old, the Alcoholic Foundation was struggling. The publication of the Big Book had been less than successful; the need for cash to pay bills was great. Rockefeller had proposed the dinner to give his wealthy friends and associates a firsthand experience of the program. Bill Wilson and the other trustees hoped this support would resolve their financial problems. Seventy-five men attended the dinner. Wilson estimated their "total financial worth might easily be a billion dollars." The dinner went well. Newly sober members of A.A. were assigned so that at least one was at every table. After the dinner, presentations began. Bill and Dr. Bob spoke, recounting their stories. They were followed by the pastor of the interdenominational Riverside Church, nationally known teacher and author Dr. Harry Emerson Fosdick, and the world-renowned neurologist Dr. Foster Kennedy. Rockefeller had suddenly taken ill, so his son Nelson took his place. After describing his father's interest, he concluded, "Gentlemen, you can all see that this is a work of good will. Its power lies in the fact that one member carries the good message to the next, without any thought of financial income or reward. Therefore it is our belief that Alcoholics

2. John B., "My Recovery in Traditional A.A.," para. 5.

Anonymous should be self-supporting so far as money is concerned. It needs only our good will." The applause was strong, and then everyone left.[3]

The disappointment was great. Why did Mr. Rockefeller have the dinner if not to provide and solicit financial support? Rockefeller did buy 400 copies of the Big Book to send to all those on the invitation list. Guests did provide some small contributions. But what was clearly more important than the contributions was raising the visibility of this new approach to treat alcoholism. Publicity from the dinner and circulation of the Book soon led to a dramatic increase in interest in Alcoholics Anonymous. For the next five years the Foundation continued to solicit gifts, but the advice that it should be self-supporting with members carrying the message to others resulted in a new standard now contained in Tradition Seven: "Every A.A. group ought to be fully self-supporting, declining outside contributions."

Concern about prestige, undue influence, and excessive power led to refinements in what is meant by being fully self-supporting. It means not accepting contributions from people, like me or family members, who are not members of A.A. It also means placing a limit on the amount a member may contribute in a single year. There are also restrictions on bequests: no bequests from nonmembers and limits on the amount a member may leave A.A. in their wills. Government and institutional grants are generally not accepted, though items where all not-for-profit organizations receive support (like tax exemption) are permissible. Income for the organization comes from member contributions and profits from the sale of literature.

To provide for smooth operation, a "prudent reserve" fund has been developed, containing the cost of operations for nine to twelve months. When the reserve declines so it is close to the nine-month limit, contributions from the membership are actively solicited and the prices of literature may be increased. When the reserve grows to be close to the twelve-month limit, the price of the publications, including the Big Book, have been reduced or left constant as expenses rose. It is rare that it drops below nine months.

People who have been active in leading a not-for-profit organization or a church generally react to what seems an absurd standard. Certainly, no business would develop such policies to restrict income. However, A.A.'s value of "corporate poverty" has worked for eighty-five years, and A.A. has continued to be focused on its mission of carrying the message of hope to the still-suffering alcoholic. A.A. owns no property; has no debt; has no

---

3. Bill W., *Alcoholics Anonymous Comes of Age*, 182–84.

endowment. It is a lean organization with a single purpose. As a leader in the church, I have often wondered if we would not be more faithful in carrying out our mission if we did not spend so much time raising money, repairing buildings, building new edifices, developing new programs, and working hard not to offend major donors.

Of course there are times when finances are challenging, but being totally self-supporting is part of the organization's ability to focus on it's purpose.

A Print Orientation in an Electronic Age

The book *Alcoholics Anonymous* has been listed by the Library of Congress as one of eighty-eight "Books that Shaped America,"[4] and *Time Magazine* placed the book on its list of the one hundred best and most influential books written in English since 1923, the year in which the magazine was first published. It has sold over 30 million copies and has been translated into more than sixty-five languages, including ASL and Navajo. In addition, numerous other books related to A.A. have been published over the years as well as more than one hundred pamphlets addressing specific topics. Today much of this printed material is available in electronic form, but the transition has been slow. We have been careful to conform to the Traditions regarding not endorsing other enterprises, not promoting our products, and maintaining anonymity. We have been even more cautious in utilizing tools like YouTube, LinkedIn, Instagram, and Facebook. To members under forty, this dependence on printed materials must seem a bit quaint. A deeper concern revolves around questions about the best way to carry the message to the still-suffering alcoholic in the younger generation.

A special concern regarding printed materials is the *Grapevine* magazine. The magazine, begun in 1944 as a monthly communication to members of Alcoholics Anonymous, is supported by subscriptions and the sale of small books composed of articles from issues over the years. For many years this proved successful, but in the last ten to fifteen years, subscriptions have been in decline. Electronic subscriptions have not yet made up the difference. Many suspect the format of printed words is simply not connecting with younger members.

4. https://www.loc.gov/exhibits/books-that-shaped-america/1900-to-1950.html#obj24https://entertainment.time.com/2011/08/30/all-time-100-best-nonfiction-books/slide/the-big-book-by-alcoholics-anonymous/

The resources from A.A. World Services (the publisher of official A.A. material) and A.A. Grapevine are extensive, emotionally moving, and have led to many changed lives; but we must discover new ways for sharing the message in our electronic age.

Media and Anonymity

Another challenge in our electronic age is the importance of anonymity. When, on Facebook, someone receives a message congratulating him or her on their "birthday," which is their sobriety date, others who are not members see the message and either ask how the recipient can only be seven years old or know the person is a member of A.A. In addition, there are online meetings of A.A. that on occasion outsiders log into, potentially breaking the anonymity of those present. This has become more challenging during the COVID-19 pandemic, when much of the regular business of groups is being done online. And, of course, Facebook, Twitter, and other social media invite people to become popular to a wider audience; a temptation some members of A.A. have used to set themselves up as examples.

The Eleventh Tradition speaks of the "need always [to] maintain personal anonymity at the level of press, radio, and film." To that phrase it is common to add "TV and social media." I find these concerns to be largely symptoms of the challenge of adapting a predominantly print-oriented culture to the new world of electronic communication. When Bill W. made the famous phone call from the hotel in Akron in 1935, he was using the new technology of the age. Technologies change, but the message remains. We are now experiencing the stress of a change in ways to deliver the message. The message of hope remains and the power of this spiritual program continues to change lives. We simply need to learn how to use the new media in conformity with the Traditions.

The Courts, Addicts, and A.A.

Central in the spiritual dynamic of A.A. is the identification of one alcoholic with other alcoholics. This understanding is contained in Tradition Three (the only requirement for membership is the desire to stop drinking) and Five (the primary purpose is to carry the message to the alcoholic who still suffers). So what happens when someone addicted to cocaine shows up and wants to participate? Or how do groups handle persons who have been legally ordered by a court to attend A.A. because alcohol and/or drug addiction were involved in their crimes? Often they come with an attitude of belligerence and defiant denial. Their presence can be disruptive to the important process of identification. How serious is this violation? What is the best way for the group to respond to these folks who are in need, but will not identify with the resources of Alcoholics Anonymous?

As I talk with members of the Fellowship I hear all sorts of stories. In many groups anyone who comes is welcome and they are allowed to figure out if they belong. In other groups, after the meeting is over someone will talk with the addict and explain that they will find appropriate help at a meeting of Narcotics Anonymous. Then there are unsettling stories in which someone introduces himself as "an alcoholic and an addict," and a member of the group interrupts him saying, "We don't talk about addiction here."

One story I love, told by a young person now in A.A., comes from her forced attendance by the court when she was seventeen. She was in full denial. She sat in the back of the room with body language that screamed out, "I do not want to be here." After a meeting, an old-timer approached her and said, "You don't think you are an alcoholic, do you?" Her reply was a sneering "no." He then took out his wallet and gave her a ten-dollar bill. "To prove you are not an alcoholic, take this to the bar across the street, buy one drink, and then leave." As she tells the story, she decided that what she could drink to prove she was not alcoholic was three beers and five shots! Obviously she did not leave the bar sober. It was a couple more years before she accepted that she was alcoholic and that A.A. could provide her the help she needed. She believes the old-timer helped her along the road to acceptance.

In the local open group I sometimes attend, one Saturday morning a mother showed up with her addicted daughter. They were not silent observers. They needed help, and they expected the group to provide it. I was in shock as the mother explained all she was doing to try to control her daughter, and then the daughter talked about her addiction. Clearly the mother needed Al-Anon, and the daughter needed N.A. With my mouth (spiritually) hanging open, I watched as the group shared their stories of alcoholism and explained the differences between alcoholism and addiction to other drugs. They talked about Al-Anon and how important it would be for the mother to attend those meetings. One member used her cell phone to look up N.A. and Al-Anon meetings nearby and shared that information. What a wonderful, loving response. I was so proud of "my group."

In my perception, we have not yet figured out exactly how to respond to addicts and court-ordered attendees who do not identify with A.A. practice is varied. But love and tolerance is our code, and as we share stories, we will develop norms.

Rigidity

At any large gathering of members of A.A., it is common to refer to those present as miracles. When we hear the stories of what life was like in the bondage of addiction, what happened, and what life is like now, the transformation is dramatic. What happened to change the speaker's life is that a power greater then she, through the Steps and the Fellowship of Alcoholics Anonymous, restored her to sanity. What happened that produced this dramatic change is nothing less than a miracle. Rarely does that power come through a magical awakening or a bolt of lightning; usually it comes as a gradual lessening of anxiety, distorted perception, and resentment, as well as an increase in self-acceptance and serenity. Though not dramatic, it is no less a miracle.

We can easily understand that when a person's life has so dramatically changed, he or she comes to feel that what happened to them is the "right way." How they understand the God they experienced, how they worked the Steps, and the advice and counsel of their sponsor together represent the true way A.A. is to be done. The Steps, which in the Big Book are called suggestions, become rules more fixed than the Ten Commandments. They may convince themselves that prayer and meditation are absolutely essential if one is to stay sober. And often they begin to preach that unless one has a belief in a deity, they are likely to slip back into the life of drinking and self-focused behavior.

We can easily understand how a person or a group can begin to believe there is only one way to work the Steps, one way to hold a meeting, one way to interpret the Traditions, or that ending the meeting with the Serenity Prayer or the Lord's Prayer is important. The staff at the General Service Office frequently get communication complaining about how other members of the group are not following what the writers believe to be the "right way." The staff write back that they are not A.A. police and that no one is an enforcer of the Traditions. They then share what other groups or individuals have experienced around the issue being addressed.

Having a single right way is indeed counter to the tradition and practice of Alcoholics Anonymous. The Steps, the Traditions, and even the Big Book are based solely on what works. Trial and error necessitates some errors. The Traditions are often referred to as a list of how to avoid mistakes previously made. There are no principles in A.A. to be forced upon a person. The inclusion of anyone who desires to stop drinking means that we have different personalities, different beliefs (including no belief in a deity at all), different cultures, different faiths, different ways of working the Steps. The diversity within the Fellowship makes uniformity impossible. Within this diverse Fellowship, rules and regulations seldom work well. Unity is based on a mutuality that comes from shared experience—that is more powerful than any set of rules could ever be.

Bill W. describes how this freedom and unity work in one of his early writings:

> Though the individual AA is under no human coercion, is at almost perfect liberty, we have, nevertheless, achieved a wonderful unity on vital essentials.
>
> For example, the Twelve Steps are not crammed down anybody's throat. They are not sustained by any human authority. Yet we powerfully unite around them because the truth they contain has saved our lives, has opened the door to a new world. Our experience tells us these universal truths work. The anarchy of the individual yields to their persuasion. He sobers up and is led, little by little, to complete agreement with our simple fundamentals.
>
> Ultimately, these truths govern his life and he comes to live under their authority, the most powerful authority known, *the authority of his full consent, willingly given.* He is ruled, not by people, but by principles, by truths and, as most of us would say, by God.[5]

Rigidity is not a new concern, rather it is a natural result for a program that saves lives. Bob P., who served as a trustee, an A.A.W.S. director, a Grapevine director, and then General Manager of the General Service Office from 1974 to 1984, addressed this concern in his address to the General Service Conference in 1985:

> [The greatest danger facing A.A. today] is rigidity—the increasing demand for absolute answers to nit-picking questions; pressure for

5. Bill W., *Language of the Heart,* 8 (italics original).

G.S.O. (The General Service Office) to "enforce" our Traditions; screening alcoholics at closed meetings; prohibiting non-Conference-Approved literature, i.e., "banning books;" laying more and more rules on groups and members. In this trend toward rigidity, we are drifting farther and farther away from our co-founders. Bill, in particular, must be spinning in his grave, for he was perhaps the most permissive person I ever met. One of his favorite sayings was, "Every group has the right to be wrong." He was maddeningly tolerant of his critics, and he had absolute faith that faults in A.A. were self-correcting.

Governance and Responding to the Challenges

For those of us who are not alcoholic and have been elected to the General Service Board of Alcoholics Anonymous as Trustees, the first year of service is filled with confusion, moments of insight, and a steep learning curve about how Alcoholics Anonymous works. All of us had attended local group meetings. All of us were familiar with the Twelve Steps and the Twelve Traditions. Most of us had served on other corporate boards and with not-for-profit organizations. Most of us had never heard of The Twelve Concepts for World Service which represent the principles designed to ensure that the various elements of A.A.'s service structure are responsive to those they serve. We had to unlearn much that we knew from our previous governance experience.

Just as the Second Tradition places authority for each autonomous group in the will of a loving God as it is expressed in the group conscience, the First Concept places the authority for A.A. World Service in the "collective conscience of our whole Fellowship." Wow! And I always thought an organization's board of trustees exercised authority for the organization. The way the "collective conscience of our whole Fellowship" is expressed is at the annual General Service Conference, which is held to conduct the business and set policy for the organization. It is indeed a different kind of organization where the authority lies with a body of approximately 130 members of A.A. who spend hours each year discussing and making decisions on agenda items that have been put forward by groups, districts, areas, and regions of the United States and Canada. The Trustees take their agenda from the actions of this Conference, placing their service to the greater whole rather than dictating to its membership in any way. Each year the first day of the Conference is spent going over reports from the Trustees regarding what they have done with the agendas from the previous year's Conference. If this sounds upside down, that's because it is. The whole structure is often referred to as an upside-down triangle. The local groups are the head of the organization, and the rest of the structure is designed to assist the groups who carry out the primary purpose of A.A.—to carry the message to the alcoholic who still suffers. The Trustees and the General Service Office do not represent a central authority.

The Ninth Tradition states that "A.A., as such, ought never be organized . . . ." After several years working with A.A. at the national level, it appears to me we have successfully honored this Tradition. I also have come to understand why being unorganized is so important. Though urged by many to build a strong central organization, Bill W. resisted. As mentioned earlier, part of the reason for Bill's resistance was that it was not necessary. Members carry a love of A.A. because it has saved their lives and brought a new life of joy and responsibility; and the penalty for enough deviation is drunkenness leading to insanity or death. I believe there is another reason for the Fellowship's continued exercise of the upside-down organizational structure. At the local level, the program is simple: one sober drunk shares with another their personal story as honestly as possible. In the sharing, the other discovers they are not alone and there is hope, and after accepting the need for help one begins a journey that leads to serenity of spirit and a meaningful life. That is the focus, the primary purpose. A strong central authority structure would take on so many distracting tasks—criteria for membership, financial security, development and enforcement of rules and procedures, publicity campaigns, development of strong relationships with other groups working in the field, and possibly even taking stances on public issues like regulation of alcohol use and criminalization of drug use. Addiction is a complex and multidimensional illness. Seeking to respond to so many issues would diminish focus on the simple task in the groups—one drunk sharing with another. The lack of organization and constantly rotating leadership prevents expertise, power, and hazardous deviation from its fundamental simple purpose.

There is a video presently going around among those who work as organizational consultants. It opens on a large group of people sitting on a hillside—picnickers. Then one person gets up and begins to dance. People stare. After a while, another comes and joins him. Then a few more. And then more and more. The point of this film? This is how movements begin.

A charismatic leader begins trying something new. Then he or she is joined by one other—the first follower, who becomes the co-leader. Slowly a few more join, and then the movement begins to grow. This growth is exponential as more and more join.

To follow the theory a little further, the movement then needs to be somewhat organized. There are two essentials: clarity of mission (purpose) and a clear criterion for membership. As the movement becomes organized, it continues to grow, but the growth become less exponential and more linear. At this stage the movement will become more effective regarding its mission.

The next step explains why this video is used by organizational consultants. Movements, after they become organized, *tend* to become institutions. They tend to become more concerned about self-preservation, finances, and property, with growing control by the leaders, and development of rules both written and unwritten to bring conformity among the members. Institutions will survive for centuries, but they are less effective in carrying out the mission, and membership growth will level off or may even decline. There is a constant need for regular renewal.

In many ways this model is a picture of Alcoholics Anonymous. A.A. begins with one charismatic leader—Bill W. He was joined by the first follower who becomes the co-leader—Dr. Bob. Growth is exponential. Clarity of mission (singleness of purpose) and a single criterion for membership (desire to stop drinking) allow the movement to be organized and continue to grow and serve the mission.

There is no evidence that the founders knew this theory; however, I believe they saw A.A. as a movement and developed the Traditions to preserve it as a movement, seeking to prevent it from becoming a self-preserving institution. Look at just a few of the ways the Traditions keep A.A. a movement:

- We have one criterion for membership—the desire to stop drinking.

- The Steps are "suggestions."

- We have clarity of mission—we call it singleness of purpose: to carry the message.

- The groups are autonomous—that's where the movement is alive.

- We depend on an undefinable Higher Power.

- A.A. is to be radically democratic, with the groups in charge.

- Rotation in leadership positions constantly brings new life and energy.

- We rightly fear a concentration of power.

- And of course there is Tradition 9: We are never to be organized.

The model asserts that successful movements tend to become institutions. It is the natural tendency. I believe the Traditions in particular are designed to keep this movement lively and focused on our purpose, avoiding the concerns of a centralized institution.

As we engage the challenges we face, there is a great temptation to seek resolution through some centralized authority. But do we really need rules and regulations beyond the Traditions about anonymity and social media, about addicts attending A.A. meetings, or about belief or nonbelief in God? Is there a right way that can be established and enforced? If we understand that A.A. is a movement, not an institution, the answer to these questions is self-evident—"no". As an unorganized, at times chaotic, movement, for eighty-five years it has remained focused on its primary mission—carrying the message of hope to the still-suffering alcoholic. And the movement is so energizing and effective that drunks are attracted to join and may even discover a power greater than themselves that is able to bring them sanity, joy, serenity, and a road of happy destiny. It is critically important that the vitality of a movement be maintained.

The way to maintain this focus, I believe, is through the power of story. At the beginning of my involvement with A.A. at the national level, I was constantly surprised about how often people quoted Bill W. It felt as if Bill was a Moses for drunks and the Big Book was sacred Scripture. Those initial feelings miss, I think, a more significant point. Citing Bill W. is less about Bill and more about a common story that members embrace, relate to, and find freeing. A.A. was founded by the sharing of personal story. When Bill proposed building hospitals and treatment centers, the members argued against this grandiose scheme. Keep it simple, they said: one person sharing his story with another. Thus the identity and spirit of Alcoholics Anonymous was born.

The importance of story is clear in the history of the writing of the Big Book. As it was being written, the group struggled over how to end the work. As important as was Dr. Silkworth's chapter affirming that alcoholism is a disease, it did not provide a structure or an identity for this new approach; it was to be used as a preface. Finally, the group decided to close the book with stories from those who had found sobriety through this spiritual program. It was already becoming the practice to exchange stories at their meetings. With this decision the sharing of stories became central, and the spirit, the identity, and the structure of A.A. followed. The sharing of stories came first; everything else followed. Thus the Fellowship itself develops a common story of suffering, guilt, despair, anger, and hopelessness that gives way to hope, surrender, acceptance, and the beginning of a new way of life. This common, though infinitely unique, story becomes the corporate identity that defines the culture of the Fellowship. The community that is A.A. was not created by research and development; the community evolved through the sharing of stories that provide mutual identification and a sense of belonging. As that identity evolved, it became clear that a centralized authority would dampen the impact of honest sharing.

First there was story. Then a spirit and culture of A.A. developed. Finally this upside-down structure emerged from the identity developed by shared stories. As we struggle with the issues we now face—God-talk, use of the Lord's Prayer, moving from print to electronic media, anonymity and social media, rigidity, issues of governance, with more to come—we have the means of resolving them: honestly sharing stories. Listening is so much more powerful than writing rules and passing motions. Sharing stories is not a very efficient way to resolve differences. A.A. is not a nimble organization; it is not meant to be. The process is rarely clear. But in the end, sharing stories will keep the focus on the singleness of purpose.

It helps to remember our common story. The fundamental issue of inclusion of all who desire to stop drinking was settled early in the life of the Fellowship through the sharing of stories. The expansion of A.A. in the US, in Canada, and ultimately into a worldwide unorganized organization in which every group is independent and each nation's organization is also independent, was developed through the sharing of stories. How to carry the message through the Big Book was finalized when the decision was made to include stories. We will not solve the challenges we face through direction from a centralized office. Rather we will share stories about our different experiences and together as a Fellowship of several million work through our differences while keeping the focus on the mission.

CHAPTER 11

To My Friends in the Church

Gratitude

FROM THE TIME I was ten years old, each summer I attended the diocesan church camp. That time proved to be life-giving. During my teen years, a time when I found myself isolated as a result of my desire for success in all things, church camp was the one time I did not feel I had to compete. I was just one of the campers. I was loved and cared for. I even remember some of my counselors. I made friends who are still friends today, and we get together at least annually. I was a different person. I knew I was loved and accepted. This experience was surely a prelude to a personal spiritual experience.

Having been ordained since I was twenty-five, my life has revolved around the mission and ministry of the church. I have been involved with small-group education. I have been involved with demonstrations for economic and racial justice. I have been involved with some fabulous musicians. I have been most fortunate to be involved with some of the most committed and talented people in our world.

The ministries of the church have provided meaning for my life. I have seen lives changed by the power of a loving God; I have seen people move from quiet desperation to joyful openness. I have been blessed to work with many groups, mostly unknown, for justice and racial equality. I was part of a significant program helping the unemployed find satisfying jobs. I have learned what it means to live as a compassionate community. I have learned how the church can be involved in effective care for those in need; how it can help those put down by our culture find meaning and dignity. I have nurtured small groups where people learned to experience God's love to grow spiritually, and I have been blessed by the academic community of theological education. I love the church. She helped me accept myself as a limited, loved human being, and she gave my life meaning through service to others. I also know we in the church are in the midst of dramatic and challenging change.

Our culture has become more and more secular, with the percentage of those who are atheist, agnostic, or no religion increasing rapidly. Religion and religious institutions are in decline. In the last ten years, those who attend church monthly or more often has declined from 54 percent of the population to 45 percent, while those who attend a few times a year or less has increased from 45 percent of the population to 54 percent.[1]

Those of us who are part of a religious institution must recognize that the challenge of secular science and anti-religious philosophy are only half the problem. We must be honest. Too much of the religion found in our organized denominations has become irrelevant, dull, moralistic, and insipid. Afraid of offending members, especially members who are generous givers to the church, the gospel gets toned down and political issues are either avoided or preached as though the preacher alone knows God's will. We rarely provide a forum that allows serious discussion of controversial issues. We want people to have a "good" experience in church. Many churches have food pantries or join with others to provide meals for the hungry. Such charitable efforts provide help for the person in trouble, but almost never address the social issues that lead to persons falling into economic difficulties. Too many people come to church believing their lives are just fine and hoping if they keep their noses clean and show up for worship, God will keep their lives comfortable. Such religious understanding is often referred to as "transactional"—we do what we believe is right, and God will keep us comfortable. There must be more than this.

Bonhoeffer's understanding of "God in the gaps" is relevant for understanding this decline. Before World War I, culturally we had a magical understanding that God could solve all problems. But as we came to understand the dynamics of economics, psychology, and therapy, God was needed to solve less and less. Guilt is resolved by a therapist. Fear of judgment after death becomes a less and less motivating reason to attend

---

1. Additional information can be found at the Pew Research Center, www.pewforum.org/data.

church. Surely if God is love, if there is life after death, there can be no eternal punishment. The result: much preaching feels disconnected from life.

In addition to tired institutions and irrelevant theology, the decline of religion has been accelerated by the abhorrent behavior of clergy and church members. The church should surely protect children, but we are confronted with scandalous and criminal sexual abuse of children by clergy.

All the religions of the world speak of all human beings as having worth and hold up visions of unity and peace, but religion too often is used to encourage conflict, and as a means for setting up members as superior while they look down on others. Throughout the Bible, the message is to care for the hungry, the poor, the widow, for strangers and children, but among a majority of the churches there is little or no support to alleviate the suffering and despair presented by the thousands of refugees to the US and refugees forced from their homes throughout the world. These shortcomings fuel criticism, disenfranchisement, and disappointment. We can understand why so many are saying that when the church becomes a means for dislike, hatred, and division, we are better off without religion.

At the same time that religion in general and churches in particular are in decline, we live in a world that is spiritually in trouble. Evidence can be seen in a multitude of examples. Extremist groups within and outside the US justify hatred and violence. The gap between the very rich and the poor has dramatically widened over the past forty years, but those in positions of power who could impact policies to support the poor seem aligned with the very rich and do nothing. The most charitable assessment of their nonaction is that they do not see the problem; they are blind and in denial. We, the richest country in the world, are unwilling to provide quality health care for all who live in this land. We are in denial about the coming disasters that may be caused by climate change. We are unable to take sensible action regarding gun violence and gun safety. The suicide rate continues to grow. Alcoholism and addiction, according to the World Health Organization, are the number one health problem for the US and Canada.[2] Even science, which has traditionally been used to advise informed group decisions, has become weaponized or ignored in order to support specific vantage points. And, not surprising for those of us involved in efforts for racial justice for the past sixty years, the sin of racism continues to corrosively subjugate one human being by another. Some of these concerns reflect systemic problems

---

2. Hazelden Betty Ford Foundation, "Addiction Research," https://www.hazeldenbettyford.org/education/bcr/addiction-research.

that oppress groups and reward biased action with political survival and longevity. Our country, and indeed many countries, have never been so divided and seemingly unwilling to take an honest, balanced stock of our affairs. Our inability to even share a common analysis of the problems we face reflects how rigid thinking patterns have become. Encouraged by political division, every individual has their own personal understanding of truth. We as a culture are divided in so many ways and are in denial about what is happening. Just when so many of our religious organizations seem to have become less relevant, we find ourselves in a spiritual crisis. The churches are needed now more than ever to be some sort of anchor.

Still, as Archbishop Desmond Tutu loves to say, "We are prisoners of hope." I love the church; I am grateful for the gifts I have been given, but we must do better. We know that beyond personal salvation, the churches and the other faiths of the world have long been committed to the principles of justice, sanctuary, and care. We welcome and advocate for the disenfranchised, for those fleeing impoverished conditions and war, and for the poor. Despite the lack of effective action, we do stand for humanity. We must be clearer messengers of hope.

While religion is out of vogue, spirituality is in. Perhaps what we need is some version of religionless spirituality in our churches, synagogues, and mosques. Just to propose such an idea raises many questions. In truth, Bonhoeffer, in his writing about religionless Christianity, raised more questions than he gave answers, as we see in this small selection from his letters from prison:

> The thing that keeps coming back to me is, what *is* Christianity and indeed what *is* Christ for us today? . . . We are proceeding toward a time of no religion at all; men as they are now, simply cannot be religious anymore. . . . If we reach the stage of being radically without religion—and I think this is more or less the case already, else how is it that this war . . . is not calling forth any religious reaction—what does that mean for Christianity? . . . If religion is no more the garment for Christianity, then what is religionless Christianity? . . . The questions needing answers would surely be: What is the significance of a church (the parish, preaching, the Christian life) in a religionless world? . . . How do we speak of God without religion? . . . How do we speak in secular fashion of God? In what ways are we Christians in a religionless world, and how can we describe ourselves and the *Ekklesia (Church).*[3]

3. Bonhoeffer, *Letters and Papers*, April 30, 1944, 91–92 (italics original).

The issues facing religion, the issues facing church, synagogue, and mosque, the spiritual crisis of our current age—these cannot be resolved easily or quickly. We cannot fix the church, and we certainly cannot fix the world. At most we seek progress. I believe that the religionless spirituality of the Twelve Steps can, even here, provide some insight into directions we might follow as we who are part of institutional religion seek to redefine organized religion to respond to our secular age.

Rigorous Honesty and Humility

People want certainty. But to seek certainty is to deny the basic limitation of human abilities. As the quote from Voltaire at the beginning of chapter 5 states: "Doubt is not a pleasant condition, but certainty is an absurd one." We have seen how the human psyche, with the preconceptions of the mind and the emotional filters of reality, is unable to discern truth. Seeking truth, therefore, is a process that involves introspection, honest participation in a community that seeks to understand, and above all, humility. And it is a process that never ends with certainty.

Still, people want certainty. In particular, they want certainty about meaning for their lives—validation of their identity, an ethic that reflects their lifestyle, and assurance of an existence beyond death. Churches, with unacknowledged or unrecognized motivation, seek to satisfy this hunger for certainty. To meet this craving for certainty, some deify Scripture as inerrant and literally true, period. Others use Scripture to prove something true without developing a clear understanding of the basis for using Scripture. Others point to the historic teaching of the church—to dogma, creeds, and agreed-upon statements of faith. There are many ways to proclaim certainty. It seems we are fearful of accepting that God is truly beyond our knowledge and that all we have is our shared experience, our shared stories, and faith.

Part of the reason, I believe, many have dismissed the church is this claim to proclaim the truth with certainty. One need only know a moderate amount of history to know how "truth" has changed over the ages. Critics find this self-assurance as evidence not of strength but of self-deception—self-deception often taught as fact. This claim to know the truth plays a central role in the churches' developing a view of us versus them. The history of Christianity's dark decades of intolerance, cruelty and compromise unfortunately tell us the results of this arrogance. At its worst it has led to witch hunts, inquisitions, and persecutions; at its best it leads to hypocrisy and denial of the reality of issues like slavery or economic injustice. I believe this claim to know the truth encourages within religion a perspective of righteousness and intolerance, the desire to control, and a spirit of perfectionism. Intolerance born of religious certainty is as old as the human desire for certainty and as destructive and ugly today as it has been in the past.

Twelve-Step spirituality invites us into a different approach to discovering truth. It begins with humility—a virtue that is cited in most religious traditions. Humility recognizes our limits and how small we are. The humble lack arrogance. Strengths can be recognized, but are often viewed as gifts. Limits are recognized without scorn or shame.

The search for truth begins with the recognition that we are limited and will never reach certainty. We all make our decisions based on preconceived notions. That is how the mind works. Humility allows us to be open to the possibility that our opinions may need correction. Humility allows us to accept self, others, and the world as they are, without having to evaluate, minimize, or exaggerate. I am who I am: I can let go of the need to be right or better. You are who you are, doing the best you can. Our world is filled with surprising joys and devastating sorrowful events. Why events happen is filled with mystery.

Clearly the problem of why bad things happen, especially to good people, is a challenge to belief in an all-powerful, loving God. But when we try to affirm the existence of God by interpreting the pain in this world as good, we risk becoming like Job's comforters, who twisted reality to defend God against Job's claim of innocence. They were indicted by God from the whirlwind.

There is a simplicity in acceptance. We don't have to interpret events or judge people; we don't have to fix everyone; we simply accept what is and discover we are often surprised by the resulting peace and, sometimes, joy. Twelve-Step spirituality begins with experience, not preconceived intellectual principles. That experience of being liberated from bondage is a spiritual transformation that comes through the liberated-humble-grateful community. As a result, we find our attention turns from self to reality that lies outside the self, and that leads easily to gratitude for all we have received. Our world is filled with mystery and beauty when we have eyes to see. Humility allows us to be amazed, to be surprised. Humility allows a spirituality that is founded on awe. We do not have to explain; we can be enthralled.

This does not mean theology is unimportant. Unconsidered and bad theology has a history of the religious forcefully seeking to impose their will on others. The wars and conflicts over what happens to the elements of bread and wine in the Eucharist is fueled by theology. On the other hand, we see the result of a truly positive theology in the work of Archbishop Desmond Tutu's Peace and Reconciliation Commission. In our own time, theology is central in the struggles over legal abortion or the human rights for the LGBTQ community. Theology is important, but we must be careful. When it is not informed by humility and compassion, it is too often used to defend one's personal opinion or to impose one's personal views on others.

Twelve-Step spirituality begins with experience. Theology is the attempt to explain experience. Experience is primary; theology is secondary. Through the lifelong process of sharing one's experience honestly and vulnerably with others, we connect. As more and more share their experience, there is a movement toward a shared understanding. The shared experience within a community that seeks truth is the basis for theological reflection. But the theological premises that emerge are personal, since the sharing is personal. They will not be for all people for all times.

The critic may argue that such an approach to theology is too subjective. We need evidence and reason, not subjective story. We need theology to give us direction for our lives. A learning I have received from the A.A. Fellowship is that stories give us direction, and they leave us free to make, and be responsible for, our choices. When the General Service Office receives questions about certain practices in an A.A. group, they understand they are hearing one side of a disagreement. They do not reply with a judgment about what is right and what is wrong; they do not see themselves as keepers of the rules. They reply with stories, with shared experiences of what other groups did when they dealt with similar issues. As we saw in chapter 7, stories have a power and provide an identity that provides guidance, but does not coerce. Seeking clear theological direction is just another version of seeking certainty. The religious story is powerful, even as it is open to diverse interpretation.

What about the Bible? Can this approach be applied in some way to Scripture? Any application of Twelve-Step spirituality to Holy Scripture will necessitate letting go of viewing Scripture as an authority containing propositions regarding ethics, cosmology, science, and all truth. I have learned from my friends in A.A. that while there is often debate about some sections, the core, integral texts serve to unify people—they serve to provide a common language and some basic instruction; they strengthen the community. When their purpose is changed to adjudicate behavior and progress, they become instruments of control rather than community. So too with Scripture, the integral story must serve to unify rather than divide. For those who have deified Scripture, accepting that Scripture does not contain all truth will be a difficult transformation. A fundamentalist approach will need to be modified dramatically. Many, however, who are not fundamentalists look to Scripture as an authority. Are there insights from Twelve-Step spirituality that provide a way for us to interpret Scripture? Twelve-Step spirituality clearly has no opinion about Scripture; it is religionless. Still, for me, the dynamics of Twelve-Step spirituality offer an approach to Scripture that is both honest and life-giving.

At the heart of Twelve-Step spirituality is the community where personal stories are shared to provide insight to the newcomer and support to the continuing members. The expectation is that the listeners will identify with parts of the stories that reflect their own lives and will refrain from analyzing and discounting parts of the stories that do not relate to them. When we look at the Bible, we find it to be a collection of stories preserved by a particular community that finds its identity as the people of God. There are two different stories of creation. There are the stories about Abraham, Moses, Deborah, Saul and David, Elijah and Elisha, Amos, Hosea, Isaiah, and Jeremiah. There is Job's story. There are stories about Daniel, Jonah, Ruth, and Esther; stories of defeat, exile, and return. There are stories about Jesus, Peter, Mary the mother of Jesus, Mary Magdalene, and Paul. There are the apocalyptic stories told by John. These stories represent a great diversity of understandings about God, the world, history, ethics, and faith.

When I read these stories as stories, I find I can identify with some, resist what some are saying, and forget others. I identify; I try not to analyze. Then these people become friends whose lives give meaning and direction to my life. Reading Scripture has become for me a little like attending a big A.A. meeting with a great diversity of speakers. In A.A., the focus is the struggle with addiction. In the Bible, I hear the voices of special friends of God; the focus is on discerning God's will. As these special friends of God become my friends, I find new insights and new experiences of grace. This approach is dynamic, does not provide definitive answers, recognizes that some stories are fiction, some myth, some legend, some bibliographic, and leaves me responsible for my choices and insights. Theology becomes a process of listening and assimilating. It begins, not with abstract thought, but with experience. Moses has a religious experience at a burning bush. Moses also struggled with the trials of leadership. Moses is my friend as I reflect on my religious experience and on the trials of leadership. In the community we share these stories about our friend Moses, and slowly, slowly there emerges a theology of liberation.

The late Bishop Mark Dyer, Episcopal bishop of Bethlehem, PA, tells a story about a man he met on an airplane. As they were in flight, the man took out a Bible and a small notebook. He would read in the Bible for a few minutes, and then he would stop and write in his notebook. Bishop Dyer inquired what he was writing. The man replied, "As I read the Bible I find particular stories and particular thoughts that reveal certain characteristics of God. I then write them down to preserve them in my mind. I have a dozen of these notebooks, filled with insights. When I die and go to heaven and see God, I will be able to say, 'I know you!'"

We can approach the insights of religious leaders in a similar way. Religious leaders from the time of Paul to the present day represent a dramatic group of special friends of God. With some I identify; with some I do not connect; some contemporary leaders I have been fortunate to know personally. All are special friends of God who challenge me to expand my thought, strengthen my sometimes-struggling faith, and give me hope.

With this approach, theology is no longer dry, abstract, argumentative, or irrelevant. Rather, it is personal reflection that emerges from experience. It is dynamic, recognizing human limitations of knowledge; it builds community; and it is humbly open to new insights. Beginning with experience, we seek understanding. The understanding, the explanation, the theology is secondary to experience. Within the community, knowing we, as limited human beings, cannot know with certainty, we take the step of faith and act, based on our experience in the community. Few passages sum up this approach to theology and action as aptly as this prayer from Thomas Merton:

> Lord, God, I have no idea where I am going.
> I do not see the road ahead of me.
> I can not know for certain where it will end.
> Nor do I really know myself, and the fact that I think I am
> following your will does not mean that I am actually doing so.
> But I believe that the desire to please you does in fact please you,
> and I hope that I have that desire in all that I am doing.

I hope that I will never do anything apart from that desire.
And I know that if I do this you will lead me in the right road,
though I may know nothing about it.
Therefore I will trust you always, though I may seem lost
in the shadow of death.
I will not fear, for you are with me,
and never will leave me to face my perils alone.[4]

Rigorous honesty begins with humbly accepting we cannot know with certainty. Such humility involves the refusal to coerce or seek to control others; it turns attention from self to the reality outside one's self. Such humility allows a spirituality that lives in gratitude for all the gifts we have received, without feeling entitled to them or condescending toward those who have less. Such humility allows us to live simply, to expect to be surprised and amazed, and to be in awe of life, others, and the world.

Mission

A second critique of institutional religion is that too often the concerns for the institution overshadow the commitment to the mission. The researcher Diane Butler Bass says it this way:

> Americans are searching for churches—and temples, synagogues, and mosques—that are not caught up in political intrigue, rigid rules and prohibitions, institutional maintenance, unresponsive authorities, and inflexible dogma but instead offer pathways of life-giving spiritual experience, connection, meaning, vocation, and doing justice in the world. Americans are not rejecting faith— they are, however, rejecting self-serving religious institutions.[5]

Alcoholics Anonymous states clearly in the Fifth Tradition that "Each group has but one primary purpose—to carry its message to the alcoholic who still suffers." This mission focus is preserved by guarding against distractions. Tradition Six states: "An A.A. group ought never endorse, finance, or lend the A.A. name to any related facility or outside enterprise, lest problems of money, property and prestige divert us from our primary purpose." Tradition Seven: "Every A.A. group ought to be fully self-supporting, declining outside contributions." Tradition Ten: "Alcoholics Anonymous has

---

4. Merton, *Thoughts in Solitude,* loc. 585 of 936.

5. Bass, "Christianity After Religion," para. 9.

no opinion of outside issues; hence the A.A. name ought never be drawn into public controversy." In any mission-oriented institution there are a legion of distractions: concerns about prestige, about how others in the area view the organization, about raising money, about property, about clout to effect change. Alcoholics Anonymous seeks to avoid these distractions by refusing large contributions and gifts from nonmembers, by renting and not owning property, and by restricting involvement with other causes or with other organizations. In the church, we add to these usual institutional anxieties with disagreements about liturgy, conflicts between clergy and musicians or assistants, regulations about membership, and more.

Now that I am retired I work as a consultant with congregations and clergy. With rare exceptions, congregations need to articulate and understand their mission. Many have mission statements running half a page, listing all the activities of the church. They operate from assumptions, not a clearly articulated mission. The clergy assume the congregation has a reasonable understanding of the faith. Members assume the way we have always done things is the right way. For many, faith is transactional—God will keep me safe and comfortable if I come to church regularly and live a decent life. To ask what is God's will for this congregation is to challenge years of practice and comfort.

One church I consulted with over a period of four years continued to revise their half-page mission statement until they arrived at this single statement: "By the Grace of God, [name of church] strives to be a community of compassion, grounded in prayer, love, and kindness." This church was one of thirteen churches in the city that participated in a program called "Family Promise" which used the church's facilities to house homeless families one week four times a year. A lot of volunteers are needed to provide food, safety, and supervision. A couple of months after they had adopted and publicized their revised mission statement, two churches in the Family Promise program withdrew because a same-sex couple with three children had enrolled. One of them was scheduled to host the homeless the next week. The Senior Warden sent an email to the vestry(the governing board) reminding them that by the grace of God they strive to be a community of compassion. Within an hour the decision had been made to extend their hospitality to the thirteen homeless children and adults enrolled in the program. This is what it means to be a community of compassion. Normally recruitment of needed volunteers took six to eight weeks; in this case they recruited all they needed in less than a week.

Without a clear, articulate, agreed-upon mission, a congregation has no criteria to evaluate programs or to discuss differences. In the words of Yogi Berra, "If you don't know where you are going, you might not get there." The lack of a clear mission means politics and controversy will provide arguments based on sentimentality, tradition, resistance to change, or embracing of change. Personal opinion dominates the discussions. With a clear statement of mission, the congregation has a framework in which to discuss differences of opinion and opportunities for new ministries. Does the decision we are exploring enhance and strengthen our mission? Too many churches are focused just on survival, which is not a mission.

The singleness of purpose found in Alcoholics Anonymous is limited and clear. To state the purpose of the church is much more difficult. There are concerns for ministry to others, for teaching the content of the faith, for justice in our world, about liturgy, facilities, and salaries, about facing illness and death. The idea of singleness of purpose seems difficult to define.

At the risk of presumptuous oversimplification, I would suggest the word "reconciliation" lies at the heart of the religious mission. The Christian ethic is founded on two laws that are found in the Hebrew Scriptures: You shall love your God with all your heart (Deut 6:5) and you shall love your neighbor as yourself (Lev 19:18). We are called to be reconciled within ourselves and to be agents of reconciliation in our world. As wounded human beings, we acknowledge that we live in a broken world, and we serve a church that also bears its own marks of brokenness. Because we are all in need of healing and cannot heal ourselves, we need a power greater than ourselves—God's Spirit—to mend, guide, and strengthen us for this task. Like the spiritual movement in the Steps, this is a movement from self-focus—concern primarily about controlling one's own welfare, reputation, status, behavior, prosperity, and comfort—to a new life formed and sustained in a compassionate community that is focused on others and on the world. We must stop depending on our own omnipotence and instead seek divine guidance. At the heart of spiritual transformation in A.A. and in the church is a movement toward openness and gratitude. When we are able to let go, ask for help, accept our fears, and live with ambiguity, we open ourselves to the love that surrounds us on every side; we become open to be part of a community of faith; we live in this world as it is and as we are, including our limitations.

Personal transformation comes through many means; most of them are probably not programmable. When we seek to provide opportunity for people to have a spiritual experience, we must be careful lest we become manipulative. In my personal experience, moments of personal transformation happen most often in groups—like the church camp experience I was given as a child and then as a teenager, like the small group multiracial group I was part of as a senior in high school, and like the small group described in chapter 6 that loved my broken friend into health. In my professional research, churches that are growing almost always have small groups as part of their program. In my experience, the most effective means for truly connecting the faith to one's personal life is through small groups.

Faith groups are something more than social gatherings. We gather in such groups to grow in knowledge and in the experience of being a compassionate community. God can be experienced in many different ways. In a small group, God is experienced through other people. Quality groups invite people to share their personal stories with confidence that what they say will be confidential. Trained leaders are important, as is training members of the group in the skills of listening. A spirit of honesty, acceptance, and humor is critical. The greater the diversity—young, old, male, female, Black, white, yellow, gay, straight, rich, poor, clever, not so clever, beautiful, not so beautiful—the richer the experience will be. These are not therapy groups; there should always be content out of the religious tradition. In my experience, it is best for clergy not to be participants. Clergy provide the content and meet regularly with the leaders. But when clergy participate the discussion changes from "What does this mean to me?" to "Am I getting it right?" Perhaps this is why Tradition Eight keeps A.A. nonprofessional. There is not time in this essay to discuss small group ministry in detail, but I do believe that the community of the church can be as supportive and transforming as the Fellowship of A.A. Not everyone is comfortable in small groups; there are other ways for personal spiritual growth and strengthening. For those who are comfortable in small groups, they can be a means for support and deep theological reflection. When the church has adopted a mission of service, a focus on building a compassionate community, and a common language for biblical and theological conversation, then the group will find sharing personal stories in the context of spiritual growing leads to personal openness, honesty, humility, and gratitude.

As individual lives are transformed, their eyes are opened, and they see the needs that surround us. Characteristics of transformed people—being accepting of limitations, being accepting of one's own pain, having the ability to share one's personal story, and having openness to new ideas and directions—lead them to form effective mutual ministries. The most effective way of ministering to those outside the church is through groups organized for justice ministries and community service, including involvement in community organizing.

What is called for in a ministry of reconciliation is personal transformation from fixer to servant and uniting with others to bring healing change to our world. Compassionate communities can exert a strong force to bring change.

Unity & Inclusion

Following the defeat of Licinius in 323 CE, the Emperor Constantine became the sole ruler of the Roman world. Now there was one emperor, one law, one citizenship for all free men. To Constantine's essentially political mind, to complete the process of unification there needed to be one religion—the Christianity he had already embraced, legalized, and officially supported. Unfortunately, from the emperor's perspective, the theological divisions in the church threatened this unity. To resolve the divisions, in 325 CE he called the first general counsel of the church in Nicaea.

This establishment of Christianity as the official, privileged, state-supported religion is seen by many today as destructive to the spirituality of the early church which depended on commitment, sometimes even in the face of persecution, rather than conformity. The established church prospered, the position of the clergy was enhanced, and the institution became—for good or for ill—a major player in social and political issues. Today, this position of privilege is declining, and many rejoice as the church must become more and more dependent on the committed.

One area of religious life deeply affected by the establishment of Christianity was adoption of the assumption that theological conformity is essential to unity. Theological agreement was certainly not characteristic of the church in its first 300 years. The New Testament is filled with controversy over the role of Jewish law for followers of Jesus, over the inclusion of non-Jewish persons into the fellowship of Christians, over how to interpret Jesus' life and being, and over the leadership of Paul versus the Jerusalem church, to name but a few examples. Controversy over the divine-human nature of Jesus, the Trinitarian nature of God, and the nature of ordained leadership continued through the four ecumenical counsels. The split in 1054 between the church in Rome and the Eastern Orthodox

Church remains to the present day. The Protestant Reformation led to a new understanding of church—a church is defined by its confession of faith. The multiplication of denominations as a result of theological differences points to the weakness of confessional churches. The efforts of the ecumenical movement to reunite the churches have been frustrated largely by the desire to reach agreement theologically.

I would suggest that we in the churches need a new understanding of unity—an understanding based on love, not doctrine. We must remember the push for theological uniformity in the church came not from the church but from the emperor Constantine, who sought theological unity to serve his political agenda to unite the Roman Empire under one religion and to be able, through the church, to impose conformity on all.

Jesus gave a new commandment to his disciples, that we love others as he loves us. That's all we need. Like the bay on Cape Cod in comparison to all the oceans of the world, we know only a little of God. My A.A. experience tells me that even given the diverse understandings of God, those small, individual experiences of a Higher Power change lives, and bring health, strength, and service to those who follow this spiritual program. Individuals work on their own concept of God, and it changes and grows as they change and grow. A little more humility within the churches—a little less assurance it has the truth, a little more love and tolerance—would go a long way toward making our churches more effective centers for healing brokenness, rebuilding relationships, and seeking justice. We cannot achieve uniformity, but we can discover unity when we are open to join in mutual service to others. It just might be true that personal growth in the church also depends on unity. Would it not be revolutionary to recognize that our unity depends on our diverse personal spiritual experience? Would it not be transformative if the church welcomed anyone who had a desire to grow spiritually? Would it not be exciting if we could join with other congregations in pursuit of a common mission? What a palpable force of spirit this would be.

Taking a cue from A.A., I suggest the nature of that unity depends on shared story, personal experience, and common mission. In the beginning, what the church held in common (and what identified the church as Christian) was the story of Jesus, the resurrection, and the record of the spread of the early church. Interpretation of the story varied. As in A.A., the sharing of stories—the biblical stories and our personal stories—comes from and generates community. Many of the biblical stories are stories of

God saving God's people: God guides Abraham to the promised land; God delivers the Hebrew people from slavery; God calls the Israelites to be the just community; God restores Judah from Babylon; God raised Jesus from the dead. Those to whom these stories relate are part of the community that retells them, recalling why we are a community. That, of course, is what we do in worship. We gather, we tell our story, we affirm our connection to the story, we reenact the story with a little bread and a little wine, and we go out changed and engaged by the power contained in the story.

Then as we share our personal stories and identify with others' stories and with the biblical stories, we are nurtured in the community of the Holy Spirit, and we become more open to others and more able humbly to learn from and serve others. The spiritual experience of humbly accepting self as I am leads naturally to acceptance of others as they are. Love and tolerance follow honest self-acceptance. Being reconciled to self opens the possibility of being reconciled to others, the first step in building a community of compassion.

As we grow in self-acceptance, we also become more aware of the need to respond to the pain in our world. At present there are many ways to be of service and to confront the brokenness of our world. We can work to dissolve polarization and model a unity based on the recognition that each person is of ultimate worth. We can embrace and promote equality among all people and reject overt and systemic racism. We can encourage open and civil discourse to bring depth and creativity to problem solving. Imagine church-sponsored groups of people with differing political views meeting together over a long period of time. When they share their personal stories with each other, and when possible they share their faith stories with each other, then new ideas for reconciliation will emerge. Similarly, when multi-racial groups and persons from diverse economic classes share their vulnerability by sharing their stories, a kind of unity will emerge, and with it plans for action and reconciliation. Through story we can identify with all people crossing racial, gender, and class lines to unite in purpose, growth, and respect. If we in the churches can discover our unity within our diverse experiences and understandings, then we can be a powerful force for reconciliation in our world.

Just as Alcoholics Anonymous, in order to carry the message of hope to the alcoholic who still suffers, developed unity, purpose, and access by having a single criterion for membership—the desire to stop drinking—so too the church can also embrace a simple criterion for membership—anyone who desires to grow spiritually—and thereby empower its mission of reconciliation to members and to those outside the community.

Jesus

As a Christian minister, I cannot discuss religion and spirituality without reference to Jesus of Nazareth. The arguments about how Jesus is related to God have raged from the time following the resurrection to the present day. Can we take a cue from the Eleventh Step: "Sought through prayer and meditation to improve our conscious contact with God, *as we understood Him*, praying only for knowledge of His will for us and power to carry that out"? Can we accept that we have different understandings about how Jesus and God are related and then seek to follow in his way?

Jesus had a dream for this world. He called it the kingdom of God. In the kingdom of God, forgiveness prevails, enemies are to be loved, children and women are honored and included, prejudice is overcome as all races and cultures are welcome, serving others is more important than religious traditions, and resistance to injustice is nonviolent. To follow Jesus is to be spiritually moved by his life and teaching and to discover ways we might seek to live the life in the kingdom. "Being a Christian is not essentially about joining a church or being a nice person, but about following in the footsteps of Jesus, taking his teachings seriously, letting his Spirit take the lead in our lives, and in so doing helping to change the world from our nightmare into God's dream."[6]

Jesus did not say, "Worship me." He pointed to God, his Father, and said, "Come, follow me. Have a meal with me. Sit and talk with me. Drink some water or wine with me." Jesus, at least as I understand Scripture and his ministry, moved outside the walls of the temple to serve the least, the lost, and the lonely. He crossed every single barrier that first-century Judaism knew—race, religion, gender, culture, and social class. He spent much time hanging out with those who were disparaged and excluded by the leaders of religion and culture. That got him into trouble with authorities, but it modeled for the world compassion, inclusiveness, and service.

The spirit of Twelve-Step spirituality affirms that understanding about God or believing in God is far less important than seeking to know God's will and having the power to carry that out (Step Eleven). In that same spirit, understanding about Jesus, believing in Jesus (which means different

6. Curry, *Crazy Christians*, xii–xiii.

things to different people) is far less important than seeking to know God's will as seen in Jesus and finding the power to carry that out. Many have questioned whether Jesus intended to start a new religion. Perhaps he simply desired to begin a movement of compassion and transformation. Religionless Christianity will be less concerned about believing in Jesus and more concerned about following in the way of Jesus.

The idea that God is love is not self-evident. The Bible is the story of God's special friends who struggle to understand the will of God. They share their stories of being freed from slavery, of being given the opportunity to establish a righteous kingdom, of captivity and deliverance, and of living under the harsh rule of the Roman Empire. There are passages that describe the love of God, but it is near the very end of the story that we finally get the insight that God is love. The experience of Jesus was an experience of God. The experience of being with Jesus led his followers to understand that God is loving, like Jesus. So finally, we reach the statement, "God is love," (1 John 4:8; see also 4:7–23), and we by the power of that love are to love others as the foot-washing rabbi loved his disciples.

For me, to say "Jesus saves" is to say that (1) I have discovered and accepted my worth as lovable because I have experienced being loved bby God through my friend Jesus and by others in my life, and (2) that I have been charged with the ministry of reconciliation which I pursue in gratitude for the love that I have experienced in the mystery of God and in the mystery of friends. (3) We are bound together in a community of compassion. These represent the three things I need most to live a full and joyful life: identity, community, and mission. I do not find this to be far distant from my friends in the Fellowship of A.A. who have accepted the limitations of their identity (I am an alcoholic) and have found their acceptance opens up the ability to carry the news of hope to those who still suffer. Our stories are so very different, and yet there is a commonality.

First Things First

Sometimes it feels very threatening to think we, the church, should give up our commitment to right doctrine, our clarity about membership, or the use of guilt and fear to bring in new converts. But we need to look clearly at the damage done by our presumption that we know the truth and that those who are not with us are less than healthy. (And that is a mild way of describing the damage often done by the church.) We need to look clearly at the impact and cost of preserving the institution, with its property, hierarchy, and wealth. We, the church, need to examine our desire for prestige, privilege, and power in the light of Jesus' temptations in the wilderness (Matt 4:1–10, Luke 4:1–12). If we do not make such a fearless, moral inventory, we will cease to exist in our secular world that no longer believes it needs the God hypothesis to solve problems. There is ample evidence that process has already begun.

I believe the model of Twelve-Step spirituality, together with the experience of those in recovery, gives us in the church some sense of security about having a God of our understanding (experience) and an openness to all who come seeking to grow spiritually. I do not believe it is appropriate to ask A.A. to somehow be a reformer for the church. A.A. has one primary purpose, and it is not fixing religion. It is the church's job to take its own inventory, and it is the church's job to let go and let God.

If we return to Bonhoeffer's reflections about religionless Christianity, we find a radical vision of a very different church. At the time he writes, neither the official Lutheran Church, nor the Confessing Church, nor the Roman Catholic Church had taken a stand against Hitler's anti-Semitism or the aggressive war. Self-preservation seemed to have taken precedence over moral witness. Thus he writes:

> The church is truly itself only when it exists for others. As a fresh start, it should give away all its property to the poor and needy. The clergy must live solely on the free will offerings of their congregations or possibly engage in some secular calling. The church must share in the secular problems of ordinary human life, not dominating, but helping and serving. It must tell men whatever their calling what it means to live in Christ, to exist for others. In particular our own church will have to take a strong line against the vices *hubris*, power-worship, envy, humbug, for these are the roots of evil. It will have to speak of moderation, purity, confidence, loyalty, steadfastness, patience, discipline, humility, contentment, and modesty. It must not underestimate the importance of human example, which has its origin in the humanity of Jesus. . . . It is not abstract argument, but concrete example which gives her word emphasis and power.[7]

He wrote in a horrific time; he confronted the church with a choice: To use one of the common sayings from A.A., "Will it place first things first, or will it continue to seek security, power, and self-preservation?"

7. Bonhoeffer, *Letters and Papers*, 203–4 (italics original).

While we may not face as radical a challenge as the Holocaust and Hitler's takeover of Germany, the question still remains: Will we place first things first? And what are those first things? Again I quote Bonhoeffer:

> Our relation to God is not a "religious" relationship to the highest, most powerful, and best Being imaginable . . . but our relation to God is a new life in "existence for others," through participation in the being of Jesus. The transcendental is not infinite and unattainable tasks, but the neighbor who is within reach in any given situation.[8]

The parallels with Twelve-Step spirituality are obvious. Religionless spirituality calls for personal transformation through the church, which itself is transformed to focus on its mission to serve those in need. To put first things first, we in the church must focus on the mission of reconciliation. We must let go of all the security and self-glorification to which we are accustomed. We must let go of the task of getting people to believe in some unprovable theology and focus on offering the opportunity for a transforming spiritual experience that will lead to acts of reconciliation in the world. All else is optional.

This type of spirituality, based in honest self-appraisal, humility, gratitude, community, and service can lead to the spiritual liberation of the individual, and to the institutional liberation of the church. We move from dogma to purpose through the same fundamental principles as are found in the Twelve-Step experience.

As a pastor, I led a congregation that built a new church building. As the president of a seminary, I led the investment of approximately 70 million dollars in restoration and reuse of seminary property. Can we reconcile the vision Bonhoeffer presents with the work of building church facilities and infrastructure? I believe we can as long as we keep first things first, and the first thing is nurturing communities of compassion where individuals find their lives renewed and where they reach out in service to others.

In addition to my ministry in regular churches, I have another experience that is perhaps closer to the picture Bonhoeffer presents. Today, I live in a very rural county in Tennessee, in the home my family has owned since 1861; it was a house for a farm on the Tennessee River. In 1942, the Tennessee Valley Authority closed a dam on the river four miles downstream from our farm. Today the home is situated on the banks of a large lake.

---

8. Bonhoeffer, *Letters and Papers*, 202.

In 1963, with helpers, I moved an old log barn down to the lakeside to serve as a pavilion and dressing rooms. Along the lake, many families who came from Oak Ridge, Knoxville, Athens, and Chattanooga built summer cabins. My mother was concerned that these folks were not going to church on Sunday mornings, as the local churches were fundamentalist and home churches too far away. In 1965, we began holding services at the barn beside the lake. Using the Episcopal *Book of Common Prayer*, my father, my brother, and a man who lived nearby led the service. There was no sermon and no collection. Because we met near the barn in case of inclement weather, the gathering became known as "St. Barnabas." Though we used the Episcopal prayer book, there was no formal connection to any denomination, and those who attend represented several different denominations, as well as none at all. It provided a place where a diverse group of people who did not know others on the lake could gather to come to know each other, to take time to worship God in the beauty of the outdoors, and to become a loving and caring community. It was wonderful for my parents, who had moved back to our home after full careers. Now that I have also moved back after retirement, St. Barnabas has allowed my wife and me to make new friends, some very close, in a new place. Over the years it has become a community that has provided support, joy, and mutual care—without clergy.

Then on February 22, 1969, an unknown person from Nashville called the Meigs County office to reserve a small room in the City/County Building for a public meeting to announce a new development—the construction of a medical waste incinerator. A state representative and fourteen Memphis investors had incorporated a medical incinerator company and had taken an option to buy a farm in Ten Mile Valley, in the northern end of our county. Tennessee had 126 medical waste incinerators. The nearest hospital produced seven tons of waste a year. The company had plans to build an incinerator capable of burning thirty to thirty-five tons a day. Tennessee had minimal regulations regarding burning medical waste and no inspection. Clearly they wanted to build this plant to burn waste from states where regulations restricted this type of facility.

After construction, the plant would produce twenty-five full-time jobs. The promise of economic development would certainly be offset by the cost of maintaining roads for the waste shipments, the decline in property values, and possible toxic air pollution. The ecological damage to Ten Mile Valley would be severe and irreparable. The profit would go to absentee owners. Clearly the Memphis investors believed they could move into a poor and politically weak rural county which would have ineffective opposition. They did not know about St. Barnabas.

Within four days after the announcement, over 200 residents of Meigs County organized to protest. In the leadership were the folks who attended St. Barnabas. Composed of local residents, scientists from Oak Ridge, an editor of *The Chattanooga Times*, business persons from Athens, medical personnel from Sweetwater, and my father, the retired Dean of Agricultural Research at the University of Tennessee. Scientists developed technical papers illustrating the multiple problems produced by the lack of regulation. *The Chattanooga Times* printed letters to the editor and ultimately an editorial calling for a moratorium on licensing new medical waste facilities until appropriate regulations could be developed. Demonstrators filled school buses, including close to sixty schoolchildren, and drove to Nashville to petition the state legislature. Officials from surrounding counties joined in the push for regulation. Approximately 500 persons attended a state committee hearing to testify to the need for a moratorium until appropriate regulations could be developed and implemented.

On February 16, 1970, the governor issued an executive order preventing the opening and operating of new commercial medical waste incinerators in Tennessee until a comprehensive medical waste plan could be developed. The company dropped its option on the land.

St. Barnabas represents a local, loving, and caring community. Formed by the love of God to bring families together, when needed it also worked for environmental justice in our world. However, to temper Bonhoeffer's radical vision, we must admit it would never have been formed in the first place without the support of traditional congregations. Though with no cost and no formal connection to any other church, it was formed by people whose faith came from their experience in traditional churches, and that connection continues to provide our shared identity and purpose.

We need all sorts of religious institutions, but we need all of them to make the main thing the main thing, to place first things first. And in church the main thing is the experience of the transforming power of God that brings personal healing to the isolated and broken, and nurtures communities of compassion that work to heal the damaged creation.

CHAPTER 12

Serenity

Spiritual Power

Jim WANTED NO PART of A.A. He thought it was some sort of touchy-feely religious cult. The use of the term "God" turned him off. He had asked God to help him control his drinking a hundred times without results. The Serenity Prayer was the proof anyone needed to know how off the tracks this organization is. "Accept the things we cannot change." Accepting, giving up, is not what Jim thought he needed; he just needed to work harder, be more disciplined, control his drinking.

Few organizations are more difficult to assess and evaluate than Alcoholics Anonymous. The membership is anonymous; every group is autonomous. There are no dues or membership fees. Every third year a membership survey is conducted, collecting only the most basic data. Given the anonymous/autonomous nature of the organization, to do an accurate survey remains a challenge. It is easy to criticize A.A. from outside. To some it appears to be a religious cult. In recent court cases, convicts have successfully argued that the court cannot force them to attend meetings of Alcoholics Anonymous because it is religious and the state may not support religion. Some social workers and counselors also refuse to refer clients for similar reasons. Other critics say that A.A. simply helps people abstain; it does not treat the underlying mental health issues that led the person to excessive drinking. Some people attend meetings for a while but then stop going. Unable to accept their powerlessness, or unwilling to get a sponsor and work the Steps, they say meetings just don't help. Many want a quick and easy solution. It's easy to criticize A.A. from the outside.

We are fortunate that current objective research affirms the effectiveness of the A.A. program. Research from the Butler Center at Hazeldon/ Betty Ford Foundation, from the National Institute on Alcohol Abuse and Alcoholism, and from the National Institutes of Health all affirm the importance of twelve-step programs for continued sobriety and recovery. On March 10, 2020, the Cochrane Collaboration, one of the most trusted groups in scholarly medicine, released a 118-page report (including thirty pages of statistics) on "the effectiveness of A.A. and Twelve-Step Facilitation Therapy." For a long time, medical researchers were unsure whether Alcoholics Anonymous worked better than other approaches to treating people with alcohol use disorder. The Cochrane Collaboration's updated systematic review, based on an analysis of twenty-seven studies involving 10,565 participants, provides the best evidence we have to date that A.A. leads to increased rates and lengths of abstinence compared with other common treatments. "These results demonstrate A.A.'s effectiveness in helping people not only initiate but sustain abstinence and remission over the long term," said the review's lead author, John F. Kelly, a professor of psychiatry at Harvard Medical School and director of the Recovery Research Institute at Massachusetts General Hospital. "A.A. and Twelve-Step Facilitation programs' interventions usually produced higher rates of continuous abstinence than the other established treatments investigated."[1] The Butler Center for Research at the Hazelden Betty Ford Foundation compiled several studies to conclude that A.A. membership and participation is positively related to improved psychosocial and drinking outcomes as well as psychological health. Based on one- and three-year abstinence rates, formal treatment combined with A.A. participation was twice as effective as formal treatment alone.[2]

I suspect it took us eighty-five years to reach this conclusion in part because we have a cultural belief that spirituality is ephemeral, untrustworthy, and not real. How can something we cannot see be so powerful? How can spiritual practice accomplish what psychologists, counselors, clergy, law enforcement, social workers, and family members could not achieve? In truth, spirituality is the most powerful force in human life. Spiritualities of control, self-aggrandizement, and conquest reap destruction

1. Kelly et al., "Alcoholics Anonymous (AA) and Other 12-step Programs," abstract, 1.

2. Butler Center for Research, "Alcoholics Anonymous."

throughout our world, while spiritualities of caring, support, and serving heal, strengthen, and enhance human life.

Among those positive spiritualities, Twelve-Step spirituality is a powerful program for freeing people from the bondage of addiction. It is estimated that this spiritual Fellowship has freed 23 million people in the United States from alcohol and drug addiction.[3] Today there are over 2 million active members of A.A. who seek to practice these spiritual principles in all their affairs. We do not need to feel shy about its being spiritual. Studies have shown that the power of this spirituality actually reprograms the brain in a manner that frees the suffering alcoholic from addiction. That the basis of this spiritual program is the pragmatic experience of what works makes it available to all—religious and nonreligious. We can be grateful that Bill W. and Dr. Bob have given us a program of such power.

I know that many who are members of A.A. and related twelve-step programs, are grateful for the gifts of freedom, integrity, and joy they have received. It seems strange to think one might be grateful for being an alcoholic, but as they live into the new life of openness, trust, acceptance, love, forgiveness, and service they find that they are on a "Road of Happy Destiny" (164). I share the following from Christine H., who wrote this shortly after her husband died.

> Loss and loneliness aren't the only things I'm feeling today. It's not even two weeks since John died so there's also a lot of numbness, a lot of not feeling at all. But I am becoming aware of a deep well of gratitude. I've had many, many years of training in Alcoholics Anonymous in how to live one day, one moment, at a time without drink or drug.
>
> I am grateful for the sober years that John and I had together. I am grateful for the easy sober laughter we shared. I am grateful for the sober spats and the sober reconciliations. I am grateful for going sober to church and for going sober to meetings together. I am grateful for our sober dinner parties. I am grateful for our sober symphony concerts and sober Red Sox games. I am grateful for the garden, a gift of our sobriety.
>
> And most of all, I am so grateful for sobriety, for recognizing that God is here with me now, and that God always has always been with me—has always been with us.[4]

3. Simon-Peter, "AA Can Teach the Church," paras. 1–2; see also General Service Office, "Estimated Worldwide A.A. Individual and Group Membership."

4. Christine H. "Nothing Will Be Able to Separate Us . . ." paras. 10–12.

I am often humbled by the faith, resilience, and gratitude I find in members of this powerful Fellowship.

Three themes run through this book: (1) Spirituality is powerful and the spirituality of the Twelve Steps, which requires commitment and discipline, is a power that transforms lives. (2) Because Twelve-Step spirituality was developed from what worked, not from philosophical or theological presuppositions, it can be beneficial to any individual who applies its principles. All of us can learn from this powerful spiritual program; all of us can benefit from practicing those portions that relate to our lives. (3) Principles defining the spirituality of A.A. can be embraced by nonalcoholic, nonaddict groups and institutions to impact their effectiveness and well-being.

Members of A.A. often acknowledge that the way of life presented in the Steps is a way that brings health, wholeness, freedom, and fulfillment. I often hear statements of belief that the process allows the person to become the person they were truly meant to be, once free of the bondage of self and alcohol. I also hear people affirm that they are able to stay sober because of the spiritual reorganization of self that the Twelve Steps brings about:

- "While I wouldn't recommend that anyone become an alcoholic, I believe that sober alcoholics living the A.A. way of life have been blessed with a gift. It's a gift that can't be bought, that can't be won in a lottery, that can't be stolen, forged, or rented."[5]

- "In great measure, we AAs have really found peace. However haltingly, we have managed to attain an increasing humility whose dividends have been serenity and legitimate joy."[6]

- "I'm free to be the person I've always wanted to be, but never before had the courage to become."[7]

- "I found a new definition of sanity. It was bigger than any definition I had heard concerning Step Two, but it was also bigger and better than my wildest imaginings. This sanity offered serenity, a feeling of wellness or well-being, possession of a center of balance from which to operate, and a feeling that my place in this world was just right."[8]

5. Dave G., "Healthy Appetite for Beer," 3:49.
6. Bill W., *Language of the Heart*, 258.
7. William J., "Man I've Always Wanted to Be," 12.
8. Doreen C., "Beyond Sanity," 23.

Twelve Steps to Religionless Spirituality

The tools developed through Twelve-Step spirituality are a resource for living far beyond just staying sober. Going to meetings, working the Steps, and getting a sponsor will allow a person to find sobriety, but continuing in the Fellowship brings strength for living in all sorts of situations.

One of my friends in A.A. was diagnosed with lung cancer when she was fifty-one. She had sobered up young as a teenager and had thirty-five years of sobriety when she received this news. She shared with me how the spiritual tenets of A.A. were essential and vital as she faced her diagnosis and grief. She did not deny experiencing fear, nor did she diminish her grief related to her possible death since she has hopes for her life and for her children who are not fully grown. But she met these with the full complement of internalized gratitude and faith. "Humility was afforded by the diagnosis itself; cancer easily creates a sense of powerlessness and vulnerability. From this place, I have strengthened the connections with my family, my community, and my personal belief in a power greater than myself." She shared with me a prayer she wrote in the first month after her diagnosis, as she worked to reconcile this new phase. While it acknowledged her fear and sadness, the prayer was characterized by gratitude for a life that she perceived as full and a desire to be useful and serve—fundamental tenets of her spirituality. It closed with these words: "I thank you for every sober breath, every vivid color, every beautiful sound—I thank you for the love so evident around me, for always granting me far beyond my fair share, for preparing me as you have. Still ever in the sunlight of the spirit, amen." The way of life supported by the spirituality of the Steps goes far beyond controlling addiction; it provides strength in the face of a fearful situation and focuses on gratitude for the love and the gifts we have received.

Alcoholics Anonymous is not a self-help program; rather it is a spiritually based mutual support program. The First Step makes this clear: "We admitted we were powerless . . ." We are unable to help ourselves. This recognition that we are limited human beings is perhaps the foundational spiritual principle. We are not even able to overcome our defects of character after we have achieved sobriety; we must have help from our Higher Power (Steps Six and Seven). I suspect the power one experiences in this program is in proportion to the ability to accept one's powerlessness. No wonder in this age, with our bootstrap/competitive culture, we have a hard time understanding the power of this spirituality.

Those of us in the church, as part of Western culture, also have a hard time understanding the power of this spirituality. Sometimes I think I hear more God-talk in A.A. than in the church. Sometimes I wonder if we in the church truly believe that God is a power able to transform our lives and, through the community of faith, to transform our world. When I teach the Steps in a class for a church group, I find most of us do not truly believe we are powerless. That First Step is really tough when one has not reached a point in their lives of surrender and willingness to go to any length to find help. I remember one response in particular by a member of a class I was teaching, "We do not approach life as though we are powerless. We analyze problems, develop resources, and solve the problem." Then, shortly after this statement I heard the same person express his frustration over the drug use of his teenage son. We in the church will find life fuller when we learn to accept that we need help, that we are not in control, and that there is a power that can bring sanity to our lives. Letting go of the need to control, the need to understand, and the need to be perfect, and by staying focused on the gift of relationships in the community that sustains us, we can find a serenity through this simple program.

I summarize this spirituality in a different, more theological way. I believe that love is the most powerful force on earth. This is, of course, what is meant when scripture affirms that God is love. In essence, the Steps are about being loved into health, loved by the God of one's understanding and loved by those in the fellowship of the church—loved when we were unable to love ourselves. Love is a power greater than oneself. It begins with the acceptance that we are not in control. We are vulnerable; we feel shame, guilt, and despair; we are unable to fix ourselves. With that acceptance and with rigorous honesty, we come to know humility and live in gratitude for the love that surrounds us on every side and the gifts we have received. Recovery and gratitude are related because they begin in the same place (freedom from the bondage of self) and have the same essence (orientation toward others). These are the dynamics of faith in the church. "We love because [God] first loved us. Those who say, 'I love God,' and hate their brothers or sisters, are liars; for those who do not love a brother or sister whom they have seen, cannot love God, whom they have not seen. The commandment we have from him is this: those who love God must love their brothers and sisters also" (1 John 4:19–21). The Steps provide an experience-based roadmap for growing in our faith; there is so much we in the church can gain by knowing and practicing them.

I am aware that some of my readers may be among those who are not in a Twelve-Step program and do not find religion easy to swallow.

Unsolicited advice is rarely helpful, so I will be brief. We are all spiritual beings. We all have a spirituality. Positive spiritualities have healing, transformative qualities, while negative spiritualities follow the dictates of the primitive mind (the amygdala), seeking safety and protection from perceived threats, be they real or not. Normally we are a mixed bag of positive and negative spiritualities. The power of our spirituality dictates our perception, our feelings, and our choices. How do we nurture our positive spirituality and allow our negative spirituality to diminish?

The lesson I learn from Twelve-Step spirituality is we need help. While small groups are not desired by everyone, in a group we learn spiritual connectedness, which requires a willingness to put aside our egos, defenses, and pride. We have to be willing to listen and learn, to allow another's opinion to change ours, to let go of being in charge and having all the right answers. In a group where it is safe to share our personal stories and where others share their stories, we find a connectedness that strengthens and heals. Our connectedness will result from, and parallel, our willingness to be vulnerable with others. The more inclusive such a group is, the richer the experience and the sharing will be.

There are lots of groups people belong to. Most do not represent a group that provides intentional spiritual formation. As a pastor of the church and not a member of A.A., I had to be responsible for developing my own personal support group. I found that when I had a member of A.A. in the group, we were much more intentional about sharing significant parts of our lives. My hope is that this essay will be helpful for anyone, religious or not, who desires to find spiritual growth through mutual support:

> Humility is the gift of joining in the spirit of connectedness with others and seeing that, together, we can create a community based on the values we all share. Respect. Dignity. Kindness. Acceptance. Integrity. Trust. Forgiveness. Truth. Fellowship. These are all the virtues and values that help to power spiritual healing and connectedness—the 'we' of recovery that strengthens us all.[9]

This is the power for all of us who are religious, for those who are members of A.A., and for those who would label themselves secular. It is truly a power for anyone.

---

9. Nakken, "Practical Spirituality for People in Recovery," para. 11.

Serenity and Peace

Dr. Bob, in has last address to the Fellowship, urged them "to keep it simple." The Big Book describes the Steps as a "simple program." Integrating the mind, feelings, choices, reactions, goals, and egos with life in a group that seeks rigorous honesty does not seem simple. How do we find the simplicity in the principles of Twelve-Step spirituality?

Wendi V. tells the story of driving with her eighteen-year-old daughter from Crystal Lake, Illinois, to Dallas, Texas, nurturing resentments against her father. Her Dad, an active alcoholic, was having surgery and needed her to be at his bedside. He had never been there when she was growing up; he had not attended her wedding; he had not helped when she divorced; he did not help as she suffered severe financial hardship. Resurrecting her resentments as she drove began to make her miserable, but she writes, "I said nothing, I called no one, and I prayed for nothing." Tempted to drink, she said nothing, called no one, and prayed for nothing. Having quit smoking, she bought a cigar, still saying nothing, calling no one, and praying for nothing. The tension mounted as she and her daughter prepared for bed. Pulling the sheet tight on her side of the bed, her toe touched something cold and hard. It was a twenty-four hour A.A. coin! She realized God was doing for her what she could not do for herself and had been all day. She shared her thoughts and with the coin in her hand had a restful night's sleep.[10]

As I read Wendi's story I thought, what a wonderful expression of this simple program—talk to someone, call someone, pray to God. Since the fundamental spiritual problem is our focus on self, seeking to heal ourselves maintains that focus. God does for us what we cannot do for ourselves. It is what we call grace. The importance of surrender, honesty, community, sharing stories, service, and gratitude are all contained in that story—talk to someone, call someone, pray to God. We are limited. We must surrender dependence on our own omnipotence. We need to ask for help. It can be as simple and as difficult as that—ask for help.

10. Wendi V., "I'll Handle This Myself," 62–65.

The Promises

There is a reward for following this rigorous spiritual program. This new life is described in a passage from the Big Book often referred to as "The Promises":

> If we are painstaking about this phase of our development, we will be amazed before we are halfway through. We are going to know a new freedom and a new happiness. We will not regret the past nor wish to shut the door on it. We will comprehend the word serenity and we will know peace. No matter how far down the scale we have gone, we will see how our experience can benefit others. That feeling of uselessness and self-pity will disappear. We will lose interest in selfish things and gain interest in our fellows. Self-seeking will slip away. Our whole attitude and outlook upon life will change. Fear of people and of economic insecurity will leave us. We will intuitively know how to handle situations which used to baffle us. We will suddenly realize that God is doing for us what we could not do for ourselves. (83–84)

These Promises are often read at A.A. meetings along with the Steps and the Traditions. I have a close friend who dislikes this practice as he worries that if we focus on the Promises, our focus remains on the self. We cannot let go of our self-focus by focusing on self-improvement. We cannot work to achieve the Promises, since they are the result of losing focus on self. For other, perhaps most, members of the Fellowship, however, the Promises hold up a vision and a promise for what life can be if one follows this spiritual program. When they first hear them, though they may be a bit skeptical, the possibilities contained here provide motivation to keep coming back. Later the Promises become a way to measure one's progress. One member described her understanding of a spiritual awakening being when one takes stock and finds that as result of the process one has become a different being. When one begins with no real connection to these promises and later finds that a good number of them have indeed come to pass, they can serve to reflect spiritual progress.

To work the Steps means to focus on our limitations, to accept that we need help, to accept our fears, to live with ambiguity, and become open to the love that surrounds us and live in the world as it is. When we are able to let go and let God, our eyes are opened, and we see the beauty of creation, the beauty and the needs of those to whom we are connected, and the possibilities for service. We move from self-focus to a healthy self-love and acceptance. As I learn to love myself in a healthy and honest way, then I am able to love others, as they are, and to serve them in healthy, not needy, ways.

Gratitude is closely connected with recovery because recovery is always a gift. We cannot heal ourselves; we need help. However, as we discover a community where we can be honest about our limitations and where we can laugh at ourselves, as we let go of our need to be omnicompetent, as we let go of our fear of failure, as we accept ourselves as imperfect, then we become more open, we accept others who, like us, are imperfect, and we discover that we have a new freedom and a new happiness. The qualities that are described in the Promises are gifts—unearned and undeserved—given to us by a power greater than ourselves. It is not so much that we have earned them as that we are suddenly surprised at how we have grown. Love and tolerance have truly become our code, and life is a new adventure with new surprises in store. Indeed, the tenets described in this book, of honesty and humility, of community and mission, of hope, gratitude, and service, seed peace, true liberation, and the capacity to love. There is such beauty in a fellowship built on personal stories, humble acceptance of our limitations, hope, and service. What a wonderful, wonderful way to live!

Serenity Prayer

God, grant me the serenity to accept the things I cannot change,
courage to change the things I can,
and the wisdom to know the difference.

Further Reading

IF ANYONE IS INTERESTED in doing further reading in this area of inclusive spirituality, I would recommend the following:

If you have not read the Big Book—*Alcoholics Anonymous*—you should read it. Much of the language is dated, but the insights that come from this community that has been to hell and back are still rich, deep, and practical.

The two books by Ernest Kurtz and Katherine Ketcham—*Spirituality of Imperfection* and *Experiencing Spirituality*—are wonderful collections of stories and insights from Jewish, Christian, Muslim, and Eastern sources. If you are a lover of stories with a spiritual kick, Katherine Ketcham's website (www.katherineketchambooks.com) has an excellent collection that she changes regularly.

Finally, I admire the work of Marcus Borg and in particular his last book before his untimely death—*Convictions: How I Learned What Matters Most*. His combination of sharing his spiritual experience with his scholarship is truly magnificent.

APPENDIX A

The Preamble

ALCOHOLICS ANONYMOUS IS A fellowship of men and women who share their experience, strength, and hope with each other that they may solve their common problem and help others to recover from alcoholism.

The only requirement for membership is a desire to stop drinking. There are no dues or fees for A.A. membership; we are self-supporting through our own contributions. A.A. is not allied with any sect, denomination, politics, organization or institution; does not wish to engage in any controversy; neither endorses nor opposes any causes. Our primary purpose is to stay sober and help other alcoholics to achieve sobriety.

Above copyright @ by the A.A. Grapevine, Inc.; Reprinted with permission

The Twelve Steps of Alcoholics Anonymous

1. We admitted we were powerless over alcohol—that our lives had become unmanageable.

2. Came to believe that a Power greater than ourselves could restore us to sanity.

3. Made a decision to turn our will and our lives over to the care of God, as we understood Him.

4. Made a searching and fearless moral inventory of ourselves.

5. Admitted to God, to ourselves, and to another human being the exact nature of our wrongs.

6. Were entirely ready to have God remove all these defects of character.

7. Humbly asked Him to remove our shortcomings.

8. Made a list of all persons we had harmed, and became willing to make amends to them all.

9. Made direct amends to such people wherever possible, except when to do so would injure them or others.

10. Continued to take personal inventory and when we were wrong promptly admitted it.

11. Sought through prayer and meditation to improve our conscious contact with God as we understood Him, praying only for the knowledge of His will for us and the power to carry that out.

12. Having had a spiritual awakening as the result of these steps, we tried to carry the Message to alcoholics, and to practice these principles in all our affairs.

The Twelve Traditions of Alcoholics Anonymous

1. Our common welfare should come first, personal recovery depends upon A.A. unity.

2. For our group purpose there is but one ultimate authority—a loving God as He may express Himself in our group conscience. Our leaders are but trusted servants; they do not govern.

3. The only requirement for membership is the desire to stop drinking.

4. Each group should be autonomous except in matters affecting other groups of A.A. as a whole.

5. Each group has but one primary purpose—to carry the message to the alcoholic who still suffers.

6. An A.A. group ought never endorse, finance, or lend the A.A. name to any related facility or outside enterprise, lest problems of money, property and prestige divert us from our primary purpose.

7. Every A.A. group ought to be fully self-supporting, declining outside contributions.

8. Alcoholics Anonymous should remain forever nonprofessional, but our service centers may employ special workers.

9. A.A., as such, ought never be organized; but may create service boards or committees directly responsible to those they serve.

10. Alcoholics Anonymous has no opinion on outside issues; hence the A.A. name ought never be drawn into public controversy.

11. Our public relations policy is based on attraction rather than promotion. We need always maintain personal anonymity at the level of press, radio, and films.

12. Anonymity is the spiritual foundation of all our traditions, ever reminding us to place principles before personalities.

A Brief Chronology

Summer 1934	Dr. Silkworth pronounces Bill W. a hopeless alcoholic.
August 1934	Ebby sobers up as a participant of an Oxford Group.
November 1934	Ebby visits Bill W. and shares his story with him.
December 1934	Bill W. checks himself in the Towns Hospital. While in Towns, Bill has his "white light" experience of God.
May 11, 1935	Bill W., in Akron in lobby of Mayflower Hotel, calls the Episcopal Church for help and connects with Henrietta Seiberling.
May 12, 1935	Bill W. and Dr. Bob meet at the Seiberling residence. A.A. is born.
June 10, 1935	Dr. Bob has his last drink.
1937	New York's A.A. group separates from the Oxford Group.
May 1938	The Alcoholic Foundation established and work begins on the Big Book.
April 1939	The book *Alcoholics Anonymous* is published.

A Brief Chronology

Summer 1939	Midwest A.A. groups separate from the Oxford Group.
February 8, 1940	John D. Rockefeller Jr. sponsors a dinner to raise awareness of A.A.
March 1941	*Saturday Evening Post* article published. Membership jumps from 2,000 to 8,000 by the end of the year.
June 1944	*The A.A. Grapevine* established.
1946	The Twelve Traditions of A.A. are formulated and published.
July 1950	First International Convention held in Cleveland, adopts the Traditions.
November 1950	Dr. Bob dies.
July 1955	At Convention in St. Louis, Bill W. turns over authority for the Fellowship to the Convention.
1957	The first General Service Board is created in England and Ireland. A.A. membership is over 200,000 in 7,000 groups in seventy countries.
January 24, 1971	Bill W. dies.

Bibliography

A.A. for the Black African American Alcoholic. New York: Alcoholics Anonymous World Service, 2018.

AA Grapevine. *The Best of The Grapevine, vol 3.* 3 vols. New York: AAGrapevine 2000.

————. *Emotional Sobriety: The Next Frontier.* New York: AAGrapevine, 2000.

————. *Emotional Sobriety II: The Next Frontier.* New York: AA Grapevine, 2008.

————. *Happy, Joyous, and Free: The Lighter Side of Sobriety.* New York: AAGrapevine, 2012.

————. *In Our Own Words: Stories of Young AAs in Recovery.* New York: AAGrapevine, 2008.

————. *Sober and Out: Lesbian, Gay, Bisexual and Transgender AA Members Share Their Experience, Strength, and Hope.* New York: AAGrapevine, 2014.

————. *Spiritual Awakenings: Journeys of the Spirit.* New York: AAGrapevine, 2003.

————. *Spiritual Awakenings II: More Journeys of the Spirit.* New York: AAGrapevine, 2010.

————. *Step by Step: Real AAs, Real Recovery.* New York: AAGrapevine, 2011.

————. *Voices of Long-Term Sobriety.* New York: AAGrapevine, 2009.

Alcoholics Anonymous. 4th edition. New York: Alcoholics Anonymous World Services, 2001.

Bass, Diana Butler. "Christianity After Religion." *Huffington Post,* November 6, 2015. https://www.huffpost.com/entry/the-end-of-church_b_1284954.

————. *Christianity for the Rest of Us: How the Neighborhood Church Is Transforming the Faith.* New York: Harper Collins, 2006.

Betsy S. "In Shambles." *AA Grapevine* (April 2020) 38–39.

Bill W. *Alcoholics Anonymous Comes of Age: A Brief History of A.A.* New York: Alcoholics Anonymous World Services, 1957.

————. *The Language of the Heart: Bill W.'s Grapevine Writings.* New York: AAGrapevine, 2002.

————. *Twelve Steps and Twelve Traditions.* New York: Alcoholic Anonymous World Service, 2018.

Bonhoeffer, Dietrich. *Letters and Papers from Prison.* Edited by Eberhard Bethge. New York: Macmillan, 1967.

Borg, Marcus J. *Convictions: How I Learned What Matters Most.* San Francisco: Harper One, 2014.

Bosanquet, Mary. *The Life and Death of Dietrich Bonhoeffer.* New York: Harper and Row, 1968.

Bibliography

Bruner, Jerome. *Actual Minds, Possible Worlds.* The Jerusalem-Harvard Lectures Book 1. Cambridge, MA: Harvard University Press, 1986.

Butler Center for Research. "Alcoholics Anonymous." https://www.hazeldenbettyford.org/~/media/files/bcrupdates/bcr_ru25_alcoholicsanonymous.pdf?la=en.

Chico C. "Building an Arch." In *Spiritual Awakenings: Journeys of the Spirit,* by AA Grapevine, 139–42. New York: AAGrapevine, 2003.

Christine H. "Nothing Will Be Able to Separate Us . . ." *Through the Red Door* (blog), July 8, 2020. https://episcopalrecovery.wildapricot.org/reddoor/9089704.

Curry, Michael. *Crazy Christians: A Call to Follow Jesus.* New York: Morehouse, 2013.

Dahill, Lisa. "Readings from the Underside of Selfhood: Deitrich Bonhoeffer and Spiritual Formation." *Journal of Lutheran Ethics,* August 1, 2003. https://www.elca.org/JLE/Articles/842.

Daily Reflections: A Book of Reflections by A.A. Members for A.A. Members. New York: Alcoholics Anonymous World Service, 1990.

Dave G. "A Healthy Appetite for Beer." In *The Best of the Grapevine, Volume 3,* by AA Grapevine, 44–49. New York: AAGrapevine, 2000.

DeMello, Anthony. *Heart of the Enlightened: A Book of Story Meditations.* New York: Image, 1989.

Doreen C. "Beyond Sanity." In *Step by Step: Real AAs, Real Recovery,* by AA Grapevine, 22–23. New York: AAGrapevine, 2011.

Eric D. "Humble Proportion." *AA Grapevine* (March 2007) 8.

Erikson, Erik H. *Young Man Luther: A Study in Psychoanalysis and History.* New York: Norton, 1958.

Ewing, Ward. *The Power of the Lamb: Revelation's Theology of Liberation for You.* 1990. Reprint, Eugene, OR: Wipf and Stock, 2006.

———. *Job: A Vision of God.* New York: Seabury, 1976.

Fitzgerald, Robert, SJ. *The Soul of Sponsorship: The Friendship of Fr. Ed Dowling, S.J. and Bill Wilson in Letters.* Center City, MN: Hazelden, 1995.

Gawande, Atul. "The Mistrust of Science." *The New Yorker,* June 10, 2016. https://www.newyorker.com/news/news-desk/the-mistrust-of-science.

General Service Office. "Estimated Worldwide A.A. Individual and Group Membership." https://www.aa.org/assets/en_US/smf-132_en.pdf.

Ginott, Haim G. *Between Parent & Teenager.* New York: MacMillan, 1969.

Haidt, Jonathan. *The Happiness Hypothesis: Putting Ancient Wisdom and Philosophy to the Test of Modern Science.* London: Arrow, 2006.

Hazelden Betty Ford Foundation. "Addiction Research: Emerging Drug Trends Report and National Surveys." https://www.hazeldenbettyford.org/education/bcr/addiction-research.

Horgan, John. "Do Our Questions Create the World?" *Scientific American* (June 6, 2018). https://blogs.scientificamerican.com/cross-check/do-our-questions-create-the-world/.

J. B. "Above All, an Alcoholic." In *In Our Own Words: Stories of Young AAs in Recovery,* by AA Grapevine, 28–29. New York: AAGrapevine, 2008.

J. F. M. "The Circle of Peace." In *Spiritual Awakenings: Journeys of the Spirit,* by AA Grapevine, 149–50. New York: AAGrapevine, 2003.

John B. "My Recovery in Traditional AA." *AA Agnostica,* March 10, 2019. https://aaagnostica.org/2019/03/10/my-recovery-in-traditional-aa/.

Bibliography

Kelly, J. F., et. al. "Alcoholics Anonymous (AA) and Other 12-step Programs for Alcohol Use Disorder." https://www.cochrane.org/CD012880/ADDICTN_alcoholics-anonymous-aa-and-other-12-step-programs-alcohol-use-disorder

King, Martin Luther, Jr. *A Call to Conscience: The Landmark Speeches of Dr. Martin Luther King, Jr.* Edited by Clayborne Carson and Kris Shepard. New York: Warner, 2001.

———. "Shattered Dreams." In *The Papers of Martin Luther King, Jr. Volume VI: Advocate of the Social Gospel, September 1948–March 1963,* edited by Clayborne Carson et al., 514–26. Berkeley: University of California Press, 2007.

K. J. C. "Mail Call." *AA Grapevine* (March 1949) 18.

Klinenberg, Eric. "Adaptation." *The New Yorker,* January 7, 2013. https://www.newyorker.com/magazine/2013/01/07/adaptation-eric-klinenberg.

Kurtz, Ernest. *Not-God: A History of Alcoholics Anonymous.* Center City, MN: Hazelden, 1991.

Kurtz, Ernest, and Katherine Ketcham. *Experiencing Spirituality: Finding Meaning through Storytelling.* New York: Tarcher, 2014.

———. *The Spirituality of Imperfection: Storytelling and the Search for Meaning.* New York: Bantam, 1992.

Lewis, Michael. *The Undoing Project: A Friendship that Changed Our Minds.* New York: Norton, 2016.

Lisa N. "As Real as I Can Be." In *Step by Step: Real AAs, Real Recovery,* by AA Grapevine, 56. New York: AAGrapevine, 2011.

McAdams, Dan P. *The Art and Science of Personality Development.* New York: Guilford, 2015.

Merton, Thomas. *Thoughts in Solitude.* Kindle edition. New York: Farrar, Straus and Giroux, 2011.

Nakken, Craig. "Practical Spirituality for People in Recovery: When We Live by Our Spiritual Principles, We Become What We Repeatedly Do." *Hazelden Betty Ford Foundation,* July 30, 2018. https://www.hazeldenbettyford.org/articles/nakken/practical-spirituality-recovery.

Nelson, James B. *Thirst: God and the Alcoholic Experience.* Louisville: Westminster John Knox, 2004.

Paths to Recovery. Virginia Beach: Al-Anon Family Group Headquarters, 1997.

Pauline B. "From Handcuffs to Hope." In *Voices of Long-Term Sobriety,* by AA Grapevine, 19–20. New York: AAGrapevine, 2009.

Pew Research Center. http://www.pewforum.org/data/.

———. "Amid Protests, Majorities Across Racial and Ethnic Groups Express Support for Black Lives Matter Movement." June 12, 2020.

"Quiet Guidance." *AA Grapevine* (May 1990). https://gugogs.org/2021/02/23/quiet-guidance-grapevine-article-may-1990-by-anonymous/.

Ralph B. "Call Before You Fall." In *Spiritual Awakenings II: More Journeys of the Spirit,* by AA Grapevine, 51–52. New York: AAGrapevine, 2010.

R. M. "An Equal-Opportunity Deplorer." *AA Grapevine* (March 1983) 21–23.

Ron N. "You Take Him." In *Happy, Joyous, and Free: The Lighter Side of Sobriety,* by AA Grapevine, 74–75. New York: AAGrapevine, 2012.

Simon-Peter, Rebekah. "15 Things AA Can Teach the Church." https://rebekahsimonpeter.com/aa-can-teach-the-church.

Sue F. "Principles Before Personalities." *AA Grapevine* (September 1994) 23.

Bibliography

Twerski, Abraham J. *I'd Like to Call for Help, But I Don't Know the Number: The Search for Spirituality in Everyday Life*. New York: Pharos, 1991.

Unamuno, Miguel de. *Tragic Sense of Life*. Translated by J. E. Crawford Flitch. New York: Macmillan, 1921. https://www.gutenberg.org/files/14636/14636-h/14636-h.htm.

Wallace, David Foster. "This Is Water." https://fs.blog/2012/04/david-foster-wallace-this-is-water/.

Wendi V. "I'll Handle This Myself." In *Spiritual Awakenings II: More Journeys of the Spirit*, by AA Grapevine, 62–65. New York: AAGrapevine, 2010.

Wiesel, Elie. *Gates of the Forest*. Translated by F. Frenaye. New York: Holt, Rinehart & Winston, 1966.

William J. "The Man I've Always Wanted to Be." *AA Grapevine* (October 1990) 11–12.

William W. *Sharing From Behind the Walls*. Newsletter. General Service Office of Alcoholics Anonymous. Spring 2012, 2.

Williams, Rowan. "The Paddock Lectures at General Seminary." *The General Seminary Quarterly* (Spring 2019) 3–4, 6–7, 11–12.

Williams, Thomas. "Saint Anselm." *The Stanford Encyclopedia of Philosophy* (Winter 2020 Edition). Edited by Edward N. Zalta. https://plato.stanford.edu/archives/win2020/entries/anselm/.

CPSIA information can be obtained
at www.ICGtesting.com
Printed in the USA
LVHW010051031021
699346LV00005B/9